CW01064738

PIZZLES IN PARADISE

PIZZLES IN PARADISE

A VET'S JOURNEY

John Hicks

Illustrated by Carol Lanfear Montgomery

HAZARD PRESS
publishers

To my parents, who equipped me for the journey,
Viv, my adored travelling companion,
and Emily and Morwenna, who skipped along the latter stages.

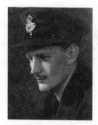

Also in memory of my uncle,
John Longton Hicks,
missing in action, 1942.

Published by Hazard Press Limited
P.O. Box 2151, Christchurch, New Zealand
Email: info@hazardpress.co.nz
www.hazardpress.com

Copyright © John Hicks 2005
First published 2005

The author has asserted his moral rights in the work.

This book is copyright. Except for the purposes of fair reviewing, no part of this publication (whether it be in any eBook, digital, electronic or traditionally printed format or otherwise) may be reproduced or transmitted in any form or by any means, electronic, digital or mechanical, including CD, DVD, eBook, PDF format, photocopying, recording, or any information storage and retrieval system, including by any means via the internet or World Wide Web, or by any means yet undiscovered, without permission in writing from the publisher. Infringers of copyright render themselves liable to prosecution.

ISBN 1-877393-05-3

Cover illustration: Carol Lanfear Montgomery

Printed in New Zealand by Keeling and Mundy Limited

ACKNOWLEDGEMENTS

In spite of the impression some readers may gain of my experiences at an English public school, life there was not unremittingly bad. My first acknowledgement is to my old English master, Peter Stott. His inspirational teaching has lived with me through the years.

I also owe a great debt to those vets who tolerated my questioning presence and gave me early encouragement to pursue a career as a veterinarian: in particular Mr Betts in Liverpool and Mike Harkness of Sedbergh, with whom I spent many happy holidays. Later in life I had the privilege of working with practice principals who were either kind, supportive or progressive and I would particularly like to mention 'Hank' de Jong of Eltham and Craig Harrison of Menston in Yorkshire.

Lastly I would like to thank my wife, Viv, for her proofreading skills, helpful criticisms and constant encouragement, and her sister, Carol, for bringing my ideas to life with her wonderful illustrations.

John Hicks
July 2005

PREFACE

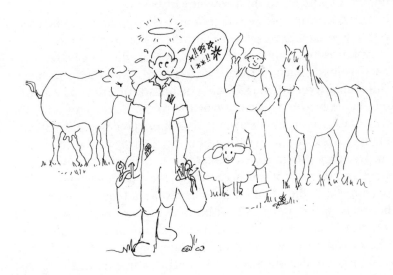

What is a vet? The public perception has been stimulated in recent years by the wonderful but historic James Herriot series of books and their widely viewed television adaptation. Recent documentaries and drama series have portrayed vets as they are trained and followed the first tentative steps of their careers.

The danger of stereotyping is ever present. Cut to a conversation at my university hall of residence. A medical student confronts her veterinary peer across the dining table.

'I can't understand why anyone would want to be a vet. I think it's sick preferring animals to humans.'

To which the rejoinder given, 'That's absurd, it's like saying a greengrocer prefers cabbages to humans', is totally appropriate.

Being a vet is not about liking animals, although it does help. For the most part it involves dealing with people and adjusting to *their* varied and legitimate attitudes to *their* animals: be they for companionship, recreation, or as a source of income.

Vets occupy positions around the world in research, industry and government departments. Clinical practice is but one avenue open to those who have qualified with a degree in veterinary science; nevertheless it is the road that most aspiring vets initially choose to follow, the one most revealed to the general public, perhaps the one about which you think you already know.

This is the story of one vet's journey to find and follow that road: twisting, rough, grotesque or hilarious as you may find it.

Apart from a couple of anecdotes, which will I hope be categorised as jokes, each incident I have described is true to memory. Unfortunately modern research is demonstrating this to be a most unreliable beast. As a child trusting to the honesty of adults it was always a mystery to me that authors could recall dialogue many years after an event without the benefit of a recording. I suspect they did as I have: created reconstructions designed to simulate the perceptions occurring in the author's memory. Well of course they did, didn't they? The resultant blurring of the lines between reality and imagination may concern the scientist, for whom objectivity and accuracy are paramount. Too often the glorious ambivalence of the English language is vandalised by him into jargon-laden submission. Conversely an enriched language enables us to express subtler nuances of feeling more in tune with the complexity of our perceptions and thought patterns. This is no scientific tract.

I apologise to any seriously scientific colleagues whom I may have offended by straying from the path of strict accuracy. Veterinarians are trained to revere science beyond all other modalities, but it is my contention that the practising veterinarian as a communicator needs skills in rhetoric and hyperbole. I may, of course, have been guilty of exploiting these on occasion. Grossly untrue statements have been made when I felt the need to rub the tip of my tongue against the mucous membrane of my cheek.

Whilst in apologetic mode: my spelling. Female readers may note that on occasions I have spelled 'she' as 'he'. Oh for the lack of a gender-neutral, singular, third person designation in these days of sexual equality! One does what one can.

To those people past and present who have shared my journey, and encounter their alter egos within these pages, forgive me should the representations or transmogrified identities not meet with your approval. No harm is intended.

CHAPTER ONE

OF PIGS AND CHRISTIANS

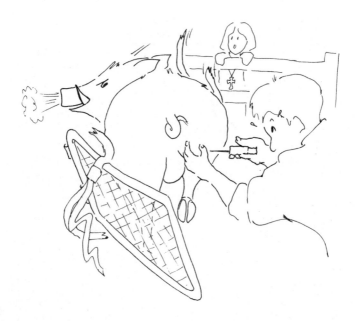

The beautiful landscapes and relaxed and friendly people of New Zealand belong to my present homeland, but my formative years were spent in Britain, parts of which still retain a special magic for me. If I cannot physically inhabit such places I file them in a treasury of spiritual homes, free to visit at whim.

Join me then as I glide over an idyllic rural England, across the undulating, sunlit downs. There below is the village enfolded between wooded hills. Church bells peal on the soft spring air. The recently-appointed vicar, released from the strictures of city life, strides out on his rounds, eager to acquaint himself with his new flock. He is a gentle soul.

Soon he falls in with a little girl being towed along by a rather large dog. In keeping with this idiom his language would have to be archaic – along the lines:

'Pray tell me little girl, what is your name?'

'I be called Petal, surr.'

'And how come you have such a charming name?'

'Well it be a bit of a long story surr, but Mummy and Daddy wanted a name from the Bible for me. They were a-looking there for names when out fell a pressed rose that Daddy had given to Mummy on their first wedding anniversary, and that's why they called me Petal.'

'That, my child, is a wonderful tale. And your dog, by what name is he known?'

'He be Porky, surr.'

'Porky?'

'Aye... He goes round shagging all the pigs.'

Barry Hardcastle related that one at the Liverpool University Faculty of Veterinary Science, perhaps around 1970. In a nutshell it parallels my own upbringing and coming of age: the ironic juxtaposition of the Church of England ideal and the cruder realities of life, of which more later.

~

Jean Sinclair's religion was more basic than this Anglican tableau, the setting more primitive. She and her husband had wrested their land from the bush. Across the river lay the Fiordland National Park. Primordial beech forest rose up: wreaths of mist draped over a sombre green, but marvellously textured, backdrop. And so it continues, ridge after craggy ridge – bush, tussock, rock and snow – falling eventually into a wild and lonely part of the Tasman Sea.

The house itself, to be blunt, was a mess – but a clean mess. Religious icons, framed tracts and Jesus figurines presided over masses of washing and ironing generated by several teenagers. This Jesus was of the type that would have made an arresting presence among the Jews 2000 years ago: milk white complexion, Viking-blond hair and china-blue robes.

As I drove up the gravelled track I had other things on my mind. Jean was now widowed, but still hanging onto the farm. I couldn't rely on much help and my immediate problem was to castrate Boris, a mature and frisky boar. This was part of what would now (execrably) be designated a 'win win' plan that Jean had adopted over the years. Use your boar as a sire over your sows for a few seasons. Everyone knows that boar meat has a taint that renders it particularly unpalatable, so once the siring is over, phase two is to remove the testicles. After a month or so without said testicles the boar taint supposedly disappears. Phase three involves slaughtering the boar and turning him into sausages; phase four, gagging them down; phase five, donating the remainder to 'friends'.

Pigs are awkward animals to handle at the best of times and in this case Boris had sole possession of an acre of bush and scrub. I immediately foresaw problems with the plan to walk him behind a gate and 'give him his injections' there. Unlike for other domesticated animals, reliable sedatives that could be injected intramuscularly into pigs just weren't around at this stage of world history. You were meant to use a vein. The textbook solution was to restrain the head with a noose round the upper jaw and secure it to a post, followed by an intravenous injection into an ear vein. Ear veins are plentiful and visible on a pig's ear, but they are fragile and positioned on a very sensitive part of the anatomy. Putting a large dose of anaesthetic into the ear of a large boar just isn't practical. The first prick elicits a forceful and lightning-fast headshake likely to snap the stoutest cord, and the hands of the would-be anaesthetist are uncomfortably close to razor-sharp tusks.

Fortunately, an ingenious trick has been devised for just this situation. Concentrated anaesthetic can be injected into the substance of a testicle with surprisingly little resentment, from where it is absorbed into the system. Once the pig is nicely comatose the testicles can be removed, simultaneously removing the source of anaesthesia, and the pig duly recovers. I had used this trick with success on smaller pigs that were induced to run headfirst into metal bins and up-ended by a stalwart farmer, thus giving me safe access to the relevant anatomy. Somehow I couldn't see this working with a 300-kilo Boris and a fifty-kilo Jean. The gate plan, however, seemed decidedly inferior.

Boris rubbed contentedly against the concrete post of the fence once he was positioned there, but it was immediately obvious that the gate, even with Jean's weight behind it and allowing for Archimedes' principle of leverage, was not going to hold him once the action started.

At this stage one of Jean's sons turned up with what seemed a possible solution. Boris was squeezed between the fence and gate with strong nylon webbing tie-downs, tightened by ratchet. The pipe gate bent ominously around Boris as the pressure was applied. It was obvious that he was getting a tad suspicious by this stage and I hastened to inject the anaesthetic solution through his scrotum, knowing that there would be no second chance.

There wasn't. At the first prick on that tender skin, Boris started to effect an escape. He crouched down, snout under the gate hinge, and with one disdainful lurch lifted the gate off its hinges. The webbing ties snapped as though they were cotton thread and Boris took off for the refuge of some trees. All was not lost; I had injected about a quarter of a dose before he was totally free. Before long we realised that he bore no malice and that, for him, this was merely a matter of personal freedom.

Accordingly my scattered assistants were persuaded to regroup and we were able to coax a by now slightly wobbly Boris into the woolshed and up a narrow race – an idea that we should have adopted in the first place (and proved entirely satisfactory for Boris' successor).

As the deed was completed, more of Jean's children and friends rolled up in a beat-up Holden and joined the spectators. This was a devoutly Christian family and I was aware that Christianity comes in many forms, but I was surprised by the directness of the question asked by a young, sweet and obviously not-so-innocent teenage girl.

'Will he still be able to have a hard-on?'

My mind raced, this was not the sort of information to be found in any veterinary textbooks of which I was aware, but vets are expected just to know these things. As I fumbled for words Jean came to my rescue:

'Not for a wee while, dear.'

Which is, of course, the perfect answer.

A month later a large package was kindly left on my desk. Our dog enjoyed the contents immensely.

CHAPTER TWO

PENNYBANK RHYMES WITH SPANK

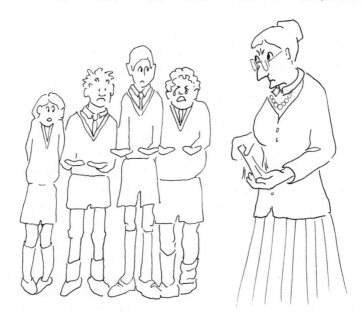

I can't remember whether they used our Christian or surnames at Pennybank primary school, but it sure as hell didn't matter. The day started peacefully enough with morning prayers, but the message never seemed to reach the zealous hearts of the teachers who controlled our lives.

For joining your o's up at the bottom, getting less than five out of ten in a spelling test and other real or imagined peccadilloes, it was the flat side of a ruler on the backs of the knees (all little boys wore shorts) or palms of the hands. For mass punishment, where most of the class were deemed to have under-performed, both hands had to be held out and, with an economy of effort, a mistress could muscularly whack her way down a whole row of cringing pupils. The psychological effect of this was more telling than the temporary physical discomfort it caused. More serious infringements merited the sharp side of a ruler across the back of the hand. An osteal clunk may lack the auditory appeal of a slap, but to the cognoscenti it is infinitely more effective.

Hurry, little boy! If you don't finish those sums soon you won't be allowed to go into the next room with Mrs Longbottom to hear the story. Look, you're the last one left and you can already hear the others shrieking at the antics of *Professor Brainstorm*. You haven't a clue, have you? No one knows why you don't understand 'simple' arithmetic. It will be a while before someone links those days of earache you suffer with deafness; longer still before you are released from your cotton-wool-world of incomprehension. Ten sums to do, some of the numbers are big. Three numbers long. There's Miss Rowe busily marking all the other children's answers. I really want to hear those funny stories.

The solution is so simple. I write down any old number at the bottom of each sum. I know they'll all be wrong, but at least I'll be able to go into the story room and hear about the professor. It will be some time before my paper is marked... Why is someone calling me out of the story room, so soon? She knows they're wrong just by looking. If you add two three-digit numbers together you can't get a five-digit answer. Wants to know why I'm so stupid. Will it be the ruler again?

Morning prayers and maths lessons. Do those nasty sums quickly and be rewarded with a nice story. Maths and divinity were my weakest subjects. I was conditioned that way.

This fifties-style introduction to academia was perhaps not untypical for many English children. We did not go joyfully to school. I concentrated very hard, but, no matter how I tried, these torments and the threat of them were daily companions.

Intermediate school was infinitely more pleasurable. The teachers were strict, but seemed to enjoy their vocation. The large Victorian house, with its spacious grounds, oozed character. There was polished oak panelling, and creaking, polished floors. An aroma of beeswax (tempered with boiled cabbage, our daily accompaniment to mince and rice pudding) pervaded high-ceilinged classrooms. Green vistas of mature trees and grass were conducive to daydreaming, because of which, no doubt, I failed to achieve my full academic potential. However, the contemplative pleasures of inner landscapes were forever mine: a priceless acquisition.

A perceptive teacher noted my deafness, and steps that I didn't fully appreciate were taken to help me to learn. What self-respecting schoolboy wants to sit at the front of the class? What little boy enjoys having his tonsils removed? Nonetheless I can remember the ice cream soothing my sore throat and my miserable earaches disappeared.

This early hospital visit was, unfortunately, but one of many subsequent brushes with institutional medicine. I was an accident-prone child and even in my veterinary career I have been too well acquainted with hospital interiors.

On one occasion I had the misfortune of holding on to a piece of timber for a builder when the skill-saw he was using kicked back and hit my left hand. I picked my thumb up from the back of the garage some five metres away and draped the rest of my mangled hand in a towel. My dear wife, Viv, ran me and a very pale builder for medical treatment.

The upshot is a disabled left hand with a missing thumb.

~

One weekend I was attending a wee Fox Terrier for a young couple and their little boy. A child in the examination room is often a recipe for disaster. The owner can't concentrate on the message you are trying to impart because half their attention is focused on the child or, if you have their full attention, it is because they have absolved themselves of all responsibility for their offspring. Then it becomes the vet's job to save him/her/them from assorted needles, scalpel blades and precious equipment as they rampage around the room. All this whilst contemplating a tricky diagnosis and communicating with the owner.

In this case I had the attention not only of the pleasant young couple, but of their very rapt young son. Throughout the consultation he continually looked from my injured hand and back into my face which he was earnestly, and obviously, trying to read. Such behaviour in an adult would have been unpardonably rude, but all was to be revealed. As the family left, the wife turned to me and apologised for Johnny.

'He's not normally like this, but we have had trouble with him picking his nose. He never stops! On the way here we told him that

16

if he carried on like that his finger would drop off.'

I doubt if Johnny ever picked his nose again, but what he thought of me was plain to see!

CHAPTER THREE

FERRY ACROSS THE MERSEY

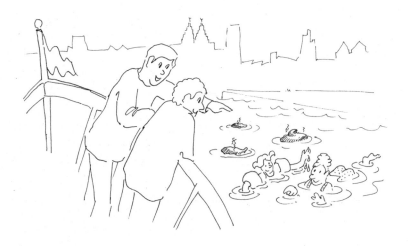

Post-war Liverpool was grim. Twenty years after the brutal bombardments, and partially cleared bombsites still blighted the city. Smoke from a million coal fires rained soot on washing. Imposing neo-classical buildings, built with the proceeds of a lucrative slave trade in preceding centuries, were neglected and coated with grime. Thick, choking smog was a frequent visitor and Liverpool was the bronchitis capital of the world. Bent old men hawked on buses, where notices expressly forbade spitting. The pavements were adorned with gobs of glistening mucus interspersed with dog turds, delivered by roaming packs of mongrels. Later I was, as a veterinary student, in a position to examine those self-same dogs euthanased and brought in by the RSPCA to further our education. It was horrifying to see that the lungs were frequently and without exaggeration: *black*. These animals had spent just a few short years on the streets inhaling soot and leaded exhaust fumes. What was it doing to *our* health?

The Mersey was present in the lives of all Liverpudlians; ship foghorns reverberated across the city through many winter nights. An occasional treat was to take the, by now famous, ferry across the Mersey to Wallasey or Birkenhead. For a child such a deviation in routine was decidedly stimulating. The seats may have been sticky but that was the norm for all forms of public transport. My mother ensured that my brother and I went through a full-scale decontamination procedure after each outing. It hadn't helped that her father was a distinguished Professor of Bacteriology.

Embarking at the docks there was always a busy scene: chains clanking, gulls screaming, children with toy windmills whirling in the breeze. The grey waters stank as they slicked between slimy brown shoals. Astern the boat, the muddy slurry muscled by the propellers glinted with petrochemical rainbows. The Mersey was in fact an open sewer, and for young children the fun was in verifying that fact. Nearing the relatively cleaner waters on the far side it was not unusual to see brave families frolicking in the floaters. We children lined the rails, avoiding the chewing gum underneath, from whence we had a more privileged view of the detritus drifting around the swimmers. 'Look! There's one heading straight for him.'

Our family would then enjoy a bracing stroll quaffing the sea air. My father was ever optimistic of the value of inhaling lungfulls of this dubious product of the Irish Sea, with its liberal lacing of industrial pollutants and decaying sea life. At this stage he was a heavy smoker, whereas we children still had functioning olfactory modalities and failed to share his enthusiasm, much to his disappointment. To this day, much as I appreciate pristine environments, the so-called 'smell of the sea' – rotting seaweed with a hint of autolysing shellfish – holds no appeal for me.

A cleaner seascape was to be enjoyed at Ainsdale Sands. On the occasional hot summer day we would drive there through the flat South Lancashire countryside, redolent with cabbage farms and bejewelled with slagheaps. The sands were firm and thousands of like-minded citizens were parked in orderly rows. Out came the canvas windbreaks and deck chairs. Adults snoozed while children disported themselves with buckets and spades. Open-topped charabancs cruised between the rows of cars...

I was never a really naughty child, but with my brother and three cousins, all boys, we were a handful.

See those grown-ups going for a ride in the open-topped charabancs. How stuffy they look, staring straight ahead. Watch their heads wobble as they hit the bumps!

Between the five of us we were able to dig quite a large trench between a row of cars and across the tracks of a hapless charabanc. The first attempt was barely adequate, but the joggled and nodding heads on the bus encouraged us to redouble our efforts.

This driver was no idiot and at the next pass chose to avoid what was, by now, a highly visible landmark. Unfortunately his evasive action bore him into soft sand. Wheels spun and he nearly stuck. A fist was waved in our direction and a distorted and angry face mouthed growly words. We had learned our lesson. The next trap had to be less visible! Suitable materials were to hand. A large cardboard box was inverted and buried to just below surface level, and we then covered it with sand.

Victory! Imagine our satisfaction when the occupants of the next busload were forced to clamber off the bus while the driver, whose body language from our safe distance signified mild apoplexy, did things with mats and spades. For the rest of the afternoon the charabanc was a distant phenomenon charting new sands where, presumably, the natives were less hostile.

Persistency and determination bring their rewards. Subsequent visits to Ainsdale Sands were a distinct anticlimax.

~

As humans we all want to know our place in society, and quite rightly have an interest in our ancestors. Mine are the usual mixture, but the more worthy of them have set standards to which I've felt I should aspire. Their example has therefore influenced my life – way out of proportion to the influence of their diluted genes within me.

This need that we have to find out about our antecedents should be an historical, as much as a genetic, quest. The more illustrious of our ancestors usually achieved their status because they were the most ruthless and corrupt members of mediaeval society. If in your genealogical research you happen to strike royal blood, rejoice in your history, but reject your pedigree!

Above all, looking backwards should remind us all that we have been the lucky generation, our lives largely unaffected by the obscenity of war.

*Stalked two ME 109s and destroyed one of them – 'jumped'
by the other but not hit. No excitement.*

This is the last, extraordinary, entry in the log book of my uncle. July the seventh, 1942. What is behind the seeming paradox of those last two words: nonchalance, bravado, understatement, ennui? We shall never know. Perhaps it was merely the truth from he who, before the war and during his precious leaves, pursued a passion for rock-climbing on British crags or mountaineering in the Alps. Excitement is exultation and freedom. Those last two words are entirely consistent from a man who had confided to my father, on their last leave together, that he got more thrills from climbing, than flying a Spitfire; and he was doing nobody any harm.

From an early age I was made aware that I bore a striking resemblance to my Uncle John. I was proud to carry his name. His mythical figure loomed large in my early childhood precisely because his loss cast a pervading shadow over the lives of my grandparents. There was no closure for them. A much-loved son reported missing. A Spitfire, modified with extra fuel tanks, perhaps the fatal handicap. No one saw what happened. Grannie and Gran never gave up hope that, by some miracle, he would one day return.

The most precious link they had with their son was an ageing Fox Terrier named, for obvious reasons, Raf. Raf had been acquired by John from a Welsh farmer just before the war. Quite a few RAF pilots owned dogs, and Raf was not the first to wait in vain for his master's return.

When I was a child we would regularly visit my grandparents, and while the grown-ups chattered above us I would enter the floor-level world of Raf. He was a dignified and occasionally crotchety old gentleman, but we had a special understanding. From that early stage I have felt an empathy with most dogs and this was certainly a factor in my later career choice.

My father's side of the family held an intriguing mix of other interesting characters. An uncle, Will, was a brilliant chemist and linguist who, between 1907 and 1910 was a lecturer in organic chemistry at Liverpool University. He had completed a PhD in Vienna. His leather-bound thesis *Über einen Fall von 'Desmotropie' beim Thiobisacetessigester* will ever remain beyond my comprehension. During the Great War he was attached to the general staff as an anti-gas expert with the rank of captain. In that capacity he was sent to Russia in 1916, was captured and imprisoned, and eventually married a white Russian, Luba – reputedly the daughter of his jailer.

It pains me to record that I always struggled with chemistry and had to re-sit an organic chemistry paper during my first year at university. Obviously the relevant genes had evaporated before they reached me.

Will's sister, Kay, gained a medical degree in 1906, one of the few women to do so in those distant years, and became an anaesthetist.

My mother's side is replete with Methodist missionaries. If religious devotion and blind faith are heritable they, too, have passed me by. My mother's father was born in India, to a missionary couple. Professor Shrewsbury, Emeritus Professor of Bacteriology in the Medical School of Birmingham University, was a true scholar. He was the author of several books, most notably *A History of Bubonic Plague in the British Isles*. It took him much of my mother's childhood to complete. Not only was he academically brilliant, but he had a distinguished war record and was a competent cricketer.

His sister, by contrast, was a check-out girl at Woolworths in Bury, which in those days was perhaps the most depressed of decaying Lancashire mill towns. She did house-keeping work in her spare time. By preference I avoid acronyms, but my great aunt Elaine could be aptly described by that psychologists' favourite: LOBNH. 'Lights on, but nobody home'. She lacked intellect, inquisitiveness, initiative: all the qualities that had made her brother great.

Elaine never married and so her nieces, my mother and her sisters, took it in turns to look after her. Once a year she came to stay with our family for a few days' holiday. It didn't take my brother and me long to realise that something was awry. We laboured long and hard to provide that missing spark in the life of our great aunt.

In those days it was possible to walk into your local ironmongers and buy a bottle of luminous paint. It wasn't for some time that luminous paint – luminous because of radioactive decay – was withdrawn from general sale. Everyone had luminous watch dials, which was very handy if you woke up in the dark, but my brother and I had more fanciful notions. By the time we had painted our picture it would have set a Geiger counter racing – not that we were to know this at the time. I have wondered if some of my health problems in later life were just retribution for this mischief.

The picture we selected was of a gruesome archaeological dig on a wild moor. Bleached skulls and skeletons lay scattered against a dismal, peaty background. Grey, smudgy clouds loured overhead. It was a miserable picture to hang on the wall of a guest-room, and an inquisitive guest might reasonably have enquired about the dubious taste of their host. But what was grim and bleak by day came alive in the dark. My brother and I had bathed every skull, every sad splinter of past human life, in thick luminosity.

We closed the velvet curtains of that large Victorian room and gleefully surveyed our shimmering work, anticipating how Aunt Elaine would interpret this new perspective of resurrection should she be called to her potty in the wee small hours. Alas, that was all the pleasure we obtained for our travail: the pleasure of anticipation. Aunt Elaine was not the sort to notice the greater detail, let alone the minutiae, of her surroundings. Less subtle efforts were required.

Aunt Elaine was fond of reading before she laid her weary head on the pillow. She didn't notice the 'dirty' dog footprints we had placed there – courtesy of 'The Wizard's Den', a shop devoted to little Liverpudlian pranksters. But she did notice when her bedside lamp, after behaving normally for a brief warm-up period, flicked off... on... off... on... off... on... This regular rhythm was not attributable to a loose connection, as she suspected. When I removed the circuit-breaker from the Christmas tree lights, all was revealed.

Aunt Elaine eventually became an unwitting but good-humoured connoisseur of false doggy doos, rubber biscuits, whoopee cushions, bending spoons and even stink bombs. She always had a lively stay at our house, and our mother refereed the worst excesses.

Elaine was placid, well-intentioned and kind. There are worse genes to share, but she never passed them on, whereas her brother's three daughters to his first marriage completed tertiary courses and a later son became a doctor. The next generation, his daughters' eight children, all obtained tertiary qualifications.

Amongst those five boys digging bus traps in the sand at Ainsdale there were two future doctors, a dentist, a successful businessman and a vet. For the last mentioned, however, it wasn't going to be easy.

CHAPTER FOUR

IT'S NOT THE LEAVING OF
LIVERPOOL THAT GRIEVES ME

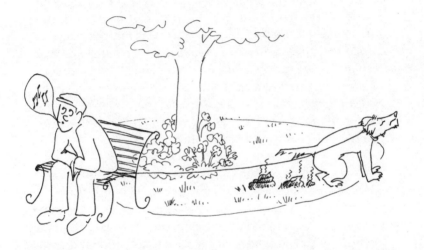

Even at a young age I was aware that this was a polluted and
over-crowded corner of the world. Once past Liverpool and its
satellites – Runcorn with its acrid pools of alarmingly coloured
chemicals, St Helens with its vast graveyard, Birkenhead with its
dilapidated shipbuilding industry – real countryside unfolded. My
parents regularly escaped at weekends to North Wales. As we went,
the flat land became hilly, the traffic lightened and the air smelt
cleaner. Soon we were in mountainous country and even then I
knew, such had been the conditioning by my parents, that I would
always seek remote places away from crowds and pollution, and
preferably amongst mountains. My uncle was not an exception; the
Hicks' family line had had a long love affair with mountains.

At home we had a large selection of books, amongst which were a
considerable number devoted to mountaineering. I consumed these

avidly, particularly identifying with F.S. Smythe, a mountaineer who ably communicated his passion for the hills. I found that I also shared his fascination with maps.

In my imagination I would start from the green plains, and follow the straggling line of a river up through the light browns, to halt firmly on one of the highest bits that represented the snowy summits of the highest peaks. There I would stop and dream, trying to picture great mountain ranges lifting far above the world: the dull walls of the schoolroom would recede, and vanish, great peaks of dazzling white surrounded me, the airs of heaven caressed me, the blizzards lashed me. And so I would dream until the harsh voice of the Geography master broke in with its threats and promises of punishment for slackness and gross inattention. If he had known, perhaps he would have left me there on my dream summits, for he was an understanding soul. (The Kanchenjunga Adventure, F.S. Smythe.)

For me, geography lessons were one of the highlights in a rather bleak academic landscape. During weekends in North Wales, long walks in the hills and mountains brought those hanging valleys, truncated spurs, drumlins and ancient moraines to life. As a family we avidly consumed books on the geology, history and natural history of the countryside surrounding the farms where my parents placed their small caravan. Each magic weekend my brother and I experienced the delights and discomforts of nights under canvas. We played with the farmers' children and 'helped' on their farms. The exquisite smell of bacon and freshly gathered mushrooms fried in butter on a purring gas stove, the anticipatory tympanic splatter of first raindrops on the tent fly, the wonder awakened by the prehistoric dolmen, the rare mystery of cow-wheat in the oak copse: these were the disparate experiences that bound me spiritually to the countryside. To this day I have retained my uncle's framed tract from the writings of the nineteenth century geologist, Adam Sedgewick:

And in the darkest hours of urban depression ~ I will sometimes take out that dog eared map and dream awhile of more

spacious days ~ and perhaps a dried blade of grass will fall out
of it to remind me that I was once a free man on the hills.

Thousands of British city-dwellers would empathise with these
sentiments. I was imbued with an intense longing to escape the
confines of city life. From an early age I knew that I wanted to be
a country vet.

~

It was in my early teens that I started to discover what being a vet
was about. Mr Betts had attended our dearly-loved family dog,
Meg, on several occasions and like most of his colleagues, then and
now, was most willing to give a young student the opportunity to
sample veterinary practice. I can still picture a stocky man with
magnificent bushy eyebrows. They had, however, mysteriously
disappeared by the time I next saw him.

Politeness forbade me asking the reason for their loss at the time,
but his receptionist gave me the details later. In short, it seems my
veterinary career had come close to starting with a bang. Like many
of his generation Mr Betts was a smoker. He was a careful and
skilled veterinarian, but I wonder what induced him to smoke when
he was performing surgery, especially when the anaesthetic used
was ether. Ether is extremely volatile and an explosive outcome
was almost inevitable.

With Mr Betts I had the opportunity to explore a totally new
world. He dealt exclusively with pets – mostly dogs and cats.
This was what veterinarians designate 'small-animal' or, more
usually these days, 'companion-animal' practice. Some practices
are predominantly 'large-animal' dealing mostly with farm animals
and possibly horses, but many are mixed, as is my current practice
in New Zealand. Individual veterinarians increasingly specialise
within practices, so that even in a mixed practice there tend to be
large-animal vets and small-animal vets. Some vets specialise in just
one species such as horses, poultry, pigs, and even, in some large
cities, cats. There are vets specialising in even narrower fields, dairy
nutrition, small-animal dermatology, canine orthopaedic surgery
and so on.

When Barry Hardcastle was bitten by a dog and trodden on by

a horse, in close succession, he opined that intensive guinea pig practice would suit him down to the ground. For all I know he could by now have acted on that facetious whim and may well be trimming guinea pigs' teeth in a Manchester suburb at this very moment.

With an ever widening and deepening pool of veterinary information there is little doubt that the move to specialisation will increase, but that does leave a dilemma for those vets servicing isolated communities. They have to be mindful of their limitations in an ever more litigious environment and still provide an effective service for all the varied creatures in their domain.

Mr Betts dealt patiently with my endless questions, gave me small jobs to do and took me with him on his rounds. These days house visits are the exception rather than the rule. It is far less time consuming if you can persuade the owner to bring the patient to you than to spend half the morning in traffic jams, only to find that Felix doesn't like strangers and is hiding under the bed. Usually it was a very large double bed with ultra-short legs. Felix was on his own territory. No one wanted to hold him properly because he scratched. Besides, they wanted to get back to watching football on t' telly. It took an age to catch, examine and treat him.

The demise of the house visit is a loss to students, because they are now deprived of the opportunity to observe the lairs of the pet-owning public. In time I witnessed the homes of Liverpool slum dwellers, London suburban housewives (maybe they were bored, but not enough to demonstrate it in front of a student), Watford film directors, and Scottish gentry. Sometimes there was time to sit down and relax over a nice cup of tea at a spotless scrubbed kitchen table – 'Get it down you while it's still hot, love'. Other abodes were a disgusting mess of filthy washing, mature chop bones, half-chewed crusts and greasy carpets, and that was before you'd raised your eyes above floor level. You could catch hepatitis merely by looking at the draining board. It was all a fascinating aspect of my veterinary education.

During my time with Mr Betts I was privileged to gain an insight into what it meant to be a professional. Never assume you know the solution to a problem: weigh up the situation by taking a detailed history – allowing for the selectivity of human memory – and make a considered diagnosis. Notwithstanding, there were conditions for which he had sovereign remedies, some of which I wish I had had the ability to record. One was his treatment of constipated dogs. This is not the favourite job of any vet that I know, aesthetics aside, precisely because there is really no easy answer.

Late on a Friday afternoon owners might retrospectively recall that he 'hasn't been for days'. Since they were coming into town to do some shopping, and he was looking a bit seedy, they thought they might bring him in for a check-up before weekend closing. What was a chronic problem has now become acute. No matter that it could have been sorted out so easily if presented earlier. This dog needs treating straight away. You are the duty vet, this is going to take an hour, and everyone else is knocking off for the weekend after a busy week. But this is a job for two people. You ask the nurse if she minds doing a bit of overtime. Being dedicated she accepts without hesitating. Half an hour later the dog is on a drip and you are administering a lubricant enema and painstakingly breaking down dried faeces filled with shards of undigested bone. No wonder the dog was unwilling to pass them. They have lacerated the double pair of gloves that you put on to start with. Think what they were doing to his rectum. That smell will be with you for at least twenty-four hours (unless you have a rotten calving to do on the way home). No finger food for you tonight. Yes, he had eaten a whole heap of cooked chop bones on Sunday. Yes, that is asking for trouble. However, to complicate matters, it may not have been chop bones. It could have been an enlarged prostate, or arthritic changes at the root of his tail. For a dog, the pathways to constipation are many and various.

The point is Mr Betts didn't seem to worry about any of this. He had an injection. I would dearly love to know what that injection was, but I suspect that, in these more circumspect days, the risk of drastic side-effects would preclude its use.

People could waltz into his evening clinic.

'Old Fergy hasn't been for days.'

After establishing the niceties of what, precisely, this meant:

'Well we could try an injection.'

'Ta, that would be great.'

People were so unquestioning. They had faith in Mr Betts. Before I put on *my* gloves today, I have to explain the procedure, get the owner to sign a consent form, and field numerous 'what if' worst case scenarios. Oh for the old days of blind faith and recklessness!

Injection duly given, I recall that the timing became critical. Mr Betts would become rather more brisk and business-like.

'It should work in about a quarter of an hour. I suggest you take Fergy up the road, you have just enough time to get to The Green. If it hasn't worked in half an hour bring him back and I'll check him over.'

Those dogs never seemed to come back. Mr Betts never had to forego finger food of an evening. However, I often wondered about the residents in the more salubrious houses overlooking The Green. For theirs was the privilege of witnessing the legacy of that little injection: hunched and straining dogs, closely watched by anxious owners, leaving voluminous deposits in their wake. Liverpool could be a shit of a place to live in.

CHAPTER FIVE

BLANCO, BRASSO, BOOTPOLISH, BULLSHIT AND LOCUSTS

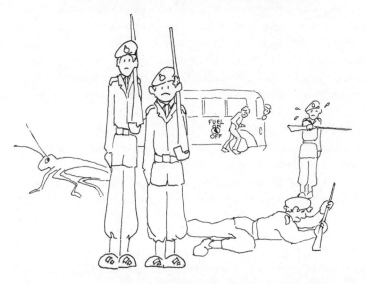

public school, pub 'lik skōōl, n. in England, traditionally, an independent, single-sex school open to the paying public with an emphasis on a classical education, physical activities and administration of discipline by senior pupils. A system of education designed to expose its recipients to the worst aspects of human nature at an early age, constrained only by antediluvian concepts of honour.

The boys queued up at the quartermaster's store for their dung-coloured uniforms ('khaki' is a euphemism). Woollen shirt, woollen trousers, woollen jacket – for the wearing of. Canvas belt and gaiters with brass accoutrements, beret with fiddly brass badge – for the cleaning of. From now on, Thursday afternoons would never be the same. We had joined our school's CCF (Combined

Cadet Force) and were destined to play soldiers. We had been sucked in by the promise of playing with real guns on the playground, rather than pretend ones. It would be a long time before we would use them for their intended purpose rather than as a prop for endless parade ground drilling, or as a punishment. Holding nine-pound Lee Enfield rifles at arm's length for the requisite time was enough to thoroughly disenchant fifteen-year-old victims with these remarkable relics of the First World War.

Even in this not-so-modern world eccentrics were accommodated, and those who eschewed violence (or were unlucky enough to have pacifist parents such as Michael Brander) were to be seen weeding the flowerbeds or cleaning the school toilets while we strutted around in our regalia. Brander carried this supposed debasement with style and, after we had had a year or two of hoisting heavy Lee Enfields around, he even succeeded in making some of us envious of his choice.

Wednesday nights were spent sprucing up our uniforms. This was not so demanding for the boarders in School House, who had the luxury of having the sprucing done for them by a fag. I had spent two years as a boarder and understood the hierarchical culture, a culture that dovetailed beautifully with army philosophy. The Duke of Wellington had declared that the battle of Waterloo (a mere 150 years earlier) was won on the playing-fields of Eton and a proud tradition of institutionalised bullying continued in many public boarding schools. What else would you expect when boys of seventeen have the power to beat and otherwise discipline their younger peers? Flashman was here. I was a late developer and I couldn't rely on Tom Brown being around when I needed him. I learned not to be noticed and developed a severe distrust of peer pressure. I learned not to be a victim; I was to be nobody's fag. That was the bottom line. I learned to distrust the establishment, for they had implemented the system. I learned to distrust organised religion, because their representatives had sanctioned it. Boys selected as prefects (usually on the basis of their prowess on the sports field) had sworn on the Holy Bible in the school chapel that they would uphold their duties with divine assistance 'God being my helper'. When one such snake-in-the-grass swore this oath on the lectern with angelic face and unctuous tones, it may have deceived the masters who had elected him to office; however,

I suspect that very few of the boys present were surprised when he was implicated in a major government scandal some thirty years later.

And that, dear reader, was the glory of the British public school system. It made you or broke you. The playing-fields of Eton spawned centuries of Empire-builders. They shaped the world. They made or broke countries. New Zealand would undoubtedly be a very different place without the influence of generations of their old-boys. Without that fiercely contested game developed at Rugby school there would be no All Blacks.

The boys in School House were as Spartans, emotionally and physically hardened, to the soft day boys. During my boarding years I had become used to ironing my trousers, wearing an uncomfortable detached and stiffly-starched collar, avoiding bullies and navigating long periods of boredom. Ideal preparation for an army career?

After a staff shake-up in the boarding school the incumbent housemaster, a minister of religion, decamped to Lahore. I had been inspired by his Christian charity on the occasion of a prolonged and alarming nosebleed following a snowball fight. 'I don't think you understand how much inconvenience this has caused me Hicks. I may even have to call the doctor.'

When the extent of mismanagement there had become known, my parents once again made me a day boy and I swapped the golden dragon badge of School House for the less imposing red porcupine of Selwyn's. This symbolically suited my frame of mind and my identification with the cult of the anti-hero. A pink hedgehog would have been even better. By this stage my two years of conditioning as a boarder were well ingrained and I felt a real sissy in the presence of my parents. Part of the survival strategy for children abandoned to such 'care', where parental access is strictly denied throughout each term, is to ruthlessly suppress any sentimental parental attachment. If you didn't your mates would sneeringly root out any such weakness in you. No one wants to be seen as a mummy's boy. Besides which, most parents encouraged their boys to be independent, disdaining overt displays of affection. Anything more than a paternal handshake would have been acutely embarrassing for both parties. Hugging your mother? Well, certainly not in public.

Looking back, it amazes me to realise how difficult it is to break down psychological barriers such as these. Eight or nine years later, at my university graduation ceremony, I was totally unwilling, even unable, to let my proud parents film the moment. Thirty years later the ceremonies for our own daughters were recorded with the love, shared pride and gratitude such events should be accorded.

Back to the uniforms. Emphasis was put on presentation. Badges were Brasso-ed, belts and gaiters Blanco-ed. Keen types played around with warm teaspoons, smoothing polish into their leather boots, and then spat-and-polished them till they glowed like mirrors. We were all keen types to start with, but for most of us the novelty wore off and some of us started to manifest signs of precocious cynicism. A prefect in School House could make his fag prepare the uniform repeatedly if the task wasn't completed satisfactorily. Or he could go the whole hog, deliberately dirty it, and make the fag repair the damage again and again and again. Power corrupts – a very valuable lesson.

The New Zealand Wool Board has since done a lot of research to remove the itch factor from wool, but as the shirts and trousers with which we were issued pre-dated the Second World War and had the consistency of tweed, those of us with sensitive skin were destined for several hours of purgatory a week. Another remarkable property of this material, shared with sphagnum moss, was its ability to hold up to ten times its own weight of water. Even when dried, a good ironing would release noisome clouds of steam. A bus full of boys in wet CCF uniforms was excellent preparation for me in later life when visiting poorly run dog kennels.

I felt the weight of history when I donned that uniform. Though we never had television at home during my school years, nor indeed in the boarding school, a defining moment in my education was an epic BBC series on the Great War. As a special treat I was permitted to watch the weekly episodes at a friend's house. Here were harrowing black and white pictures of trench warfare. Miserable, haunted, smeared faces peered out of desolate, body-littered mudscapes. I felt doubly for those soldiers in their damp, itchy and vermin-infested clothing.

Apart from the parade ground drilling, we did learn a few skills in the CCF. Unpleasant experiences can be enlightening and there were occasions when we positively enjoyed ourselves and actually pulled a trigger, or did a field exercise. One such was the annual 'Gallipoli Shield' competition contested by the six houses.

On the day, each house embussed at 0800 hrs for the trip to the chosen area. There we duly leopard crawled, completed right flanking attacks, had blanks fired over our heads, did an assault course, stripped and assembled Bren guns – the works. Day's end (1630 hrs) witnessed teams of tired boys slowly assembling beside their respective buses. At this juncture I happened to notice that some of the buses had a tap recessed into the side panel with a clear label << Fuel Line – on/off >>. To schoolboys with anti-establishment leanings this seemed like an open invitation. My friend John Watson had a mechanical bent (and has subsequently enjoyed a distinguished career in aeronautical engineering) and his curiosity was aroused. While I acted as decoy and lookout, and the harried masters checked their registers for the slow and indolent, John investigated. With sublime subtlety he spurned the opportunity to turn the tap completely off. His innate empiricism drove him to see what would happen if the tap was turned to a *three-quarters* position. That bus was carrying the School House boys.

Soon after the Selwyn's bus started along the twisting lane for home, John's question was answered. Boys in the back of our bus, who had no knowledge of what had preceded their observations, reported that the bus behind was having trouble keeping up. Sometimes it seemed to surge forwards and nearly catch us up, but increasingly it fell behind and eventually it was a mere dot in the distance as we merrily proceeded on our way. As John and I glowed with the inner satisfaction of a job well done it did dawn on us that the ramifications, should we be rumbled, would be severe. We had the discipline (courtesy of CCF training) to keep our lips sealed, as they have been till this day.

Meanwhile, on the School House bus, tired and hungry boys were starting to realise they would be late for tea. Even army discipline has its limits and on that bus they must have been breached. As a result Gallipoli Shield points were deducted for poor behaviour. Anyone looking in the school record books will now know the true story behind Selwyn's wresting of the Gallipoli Shield from School House in 1965. Life is so unfair.

~

Under sufferance, there was another uniform that I had to wear, this time on Saturday afternoons. That was when the woggle and neckerchief came out and we repaired to the Scout den. I tolerated all the badge work because at the end of the school year this troop indulged in some seriously good, and occasionally bad, adventures. With them I had canoed down the Ribble in full spate, been spat on by a drunken Irish nationalist in Dublin (it was not a good idea to wear a Scout uniform in Eire in those days and our leaders shouldn't have been so indiscreet as to fly the Union Jack at our campsite) and enjoyed a delightful camping and backpacking trip in the Austrian Alps. Our next trip led by that unctuous-toned prefect, the aforementioned snake-in-the-grass, was to be a seriously bad one. Once again we returned to Austria.

Under immature leadership our band of teenage boys disintegrated into factions. This was to be a fascinating reconstruction of *Lord of the Flies*, set in an alpine wonderland. The fact that there were no fatalities was more a matter of luck than good management.

A line of sixteen boys laden with packs and tents struggled up towards the pass. It was hot. Hard to credit the news relayed to us by a descending climbing party. They seemed amazed that we intended to cross the large snowfield on the other side. It was steep and very icy. No rope! No ice axes! We should take heed of their warnings. We did. Snake spotted an interesting-looking side-track we could follow. The map and decision-making were solely entrusted to him, by him, and to his prefect chums. Their experience was meagre, more meagre than many others in the party, but they owed their positions of power to parents willing to sacrifice evenings to their advancement: bridge nights with the headmaster. That is how the system works. The seeds of many disasters before and since Gallipoli were sown on the back of corrupt privilege.

And so we trudged haplessly down an ever narrowing track. There was a sign in German, set below a skull-and-crossbones. The sinister symbolism is international, but unfortunately only one of our party had studied German. Haltingly, at Snake's request, he translated, 'On pain of death, keep to the left side of the valley'. It sounded convincing, we didn't want to detect any bullshit. It would have been such a fag climbing back up the valley, and ignobly slinking past the hotel we had theatrically trooped by that morning.

Then we were all-conquering heroes, but our very inexperience would have been flagged to any true men of the mountains by the Hollywood of bright new billies and bedrolls barnacled to the outside of our packs.

On we went, over increasingly difficult ground, keeping left. Keen types scented victory. They needed to lead at all costs. As long as they are first to camp, they have won. Tough that their victory expends all their energy and they have to loll around recovering whilst lesser boys cook and clean.

They were well ahead of our main bunch and had now arrived at the edge of a rather large cliff, down which two of them proceeded to lose their packs. Down they bounced, spewing contents as they went, including all our money and travellers cheques. Suddenly these front-runners lost the will to press on and decided to wait for us. But we never reached them. Stopping was their first sensible decision, for down that very cliff three members of the Austrian army had recently plummeted to their deaths, leading to the erection of a sign on the track which, in fact, translated as, 'On pain of death, *do not go beyond this point*'. Sometimes getting it half right is not good enough.

Meanwhile, further back, on the left hand side of the valley (is that looking up or down?) I thought I had found a way down a rather awkward section. I was spread-eagled in an exposed position. Beneath my feet a twelve-foot drop onto a steep scree slope. The trouble was my confounded rucksack. Forty pounds is a considerable handicap. It slowly dawned on me that I was in a position from which I could not advance or retreat. I was going to have to let go. My legs shook, my hand-holds slackened. Why linger? Consciously I consigned myself to my fate and peeled backwards off the face. I was prepared for the worst. In a blurring second or two there concentrated an overpoweringly malign, regretful flashback of my short life.

My pack cushioned the first impact on the scree. I somersaulted and lay winded on the slope, mercifully intact, apart from a gashed forehead. Apparently it looked spectacular, but I was too drained to acknowledge the salutations of my peers. The horror of those few seconds would play back in my mind for a while yet.

Shocked but relieved, our group spent a wet and uncomfortable night on a steep slope. Unable to pitch our tents we tied them to trees to prevent us sliding into a rushing gorge. Sheepishly the leading group trudged back up to us and appeared out of the damp gloom to relay their tale of woe.

In the morning I glimpsed the dainty elegance of a chamois across the stream, and she was gone; a bright jewel in a tarnished ordeal.

We had been very stupid and, later on, Snake and his lieutenants were suitably upbraided by local officials. They did not appreciate helping to search the area at the base of the precipice for the equipment these silly boys had lost: ground that naturally held more poignant significance for them. I almost felt sorry for Snake, but his ego was more than a match for this challenge and he appeared unchastened by the ordeal. The makings of his political career were already in train.

A bedraggled party of wet, bruised and, in my case, bloody boys were offered hospitality in the hotel. I rather hoped that the pretty waitress would attend to my war wounds, but she obviously hadn't read any romantic Edwardian literature about wounded heroes and showed no interest in my plight.

All in all I rated it a capital learning experience, far more valuable than dressing up as soldiers on the parade ground.

~

In my later school years I was fortunate enough to become interested in my school subjects and my academic performance lifted to a level where it was conceivable that I might, with application, achieve my objective of being a vet. Perhaps it was the introduction of biology to the syllabus that fired me. Mr Swift had my attention within minutes of explaining the glories of photosynthesis. How life on this planet as we know it depends ultimately on this tiny chlorophyll molecule, present in all green plants, to fix the energy of the sun and manufacture chemicals that sustain plant growth.

'Our ancestors worshipped the sun, boys, and it strikes me that they had a lot more sense than us!'

Yet Mr Swift, not an hour earlier, had been singing hymns with the other masters at our daily chapel service. What had happened to his 'faith'? The attraction of the sciences was that they were not based upon faith. Rote learning was secondary to the development of a questioning and investigative attitude. Since Junior school days, when we had compulsorily to learn a hymn for our weekend homework, I had had great difficulty assimilating unexplained – perhaps inexplicable – mumbo-jumbo. To be fair I must admit that it wasn't always a hymn. It might be a psalm.

One weekend we were allowed a special privilege. On Monday morning all we would have to do was write out any two consecutive verses that we had memorised from the Bible. Many boys learned that weekend that the verses adjacent to 'Jesus wept' are both relatively long. I 'cleverly' plumped for two verses with a shorter combined length. It took me a long time to find them.

Mr Swift's surprising utterance lifted a great weight from my shoulders. So some adults other than my parents (parental opinion being of little moment at this stage of life) shared my growing doubts! Perhaps it didn't matter that I had declined to be confirmed into the Anglican Church after all. I had known that I couldn't live up to the expected standards. I had also known that many of those taking their vows were demonstrably unable to adhere to them; yea, though it troubled them not. Henceforth I would just have to go hungry and thirsty at Holy Communion while the exalted ones ate Christ's body and drank His blood.

Our homework assignments were also becoming more interesting. One holiday the biology class were each allocated locusts and briefly instructed as to feeding and housing (the latter to be manufactured at the boy's initiative, with parental supervision if they were canny – mine weren't). This Malthusian experiment must have caused severe consternation in many households apart from my own. Finding the lawn clippings on which to feed the burgeoning hordes was not too much of a problem over the summer holidays, but delivering it to them was. Lightning-fast reflexes were needed as that Heath-Robinson door required opening ever wider and more frequently. Eyes focused on the grotesque, fizzing adults tended to neglect the athletic offspring of a multitude of incestuous couplings. Given the slightest opportunity they leapt out of the confines of their makeshift homes and embarked on hazardous journeys of discovery. It was quite surprising where they or their crunchy carcases could materialise. My mother wasn't the only one who was not amused, but then her sensibilities may have been primed by a previous experiment with stick insects.

By nature stick insects are more sedate and less flighty than their locust cousins, but their propensity to eat portions of each other, if underfed in overcrowded situations, registered very closely as a disgust factor.

It is fortunate that the vagaries of English weather are inimical to locust physiology, which was why we had been instructed to keep them indoors, but when they've outgrown their welcome in the parental home, what then?

At the heart of many English parks there is that throw-back to Crystal Palace and Victorian enthusiasm – a large green house. One day an inquisitive colleague took it upon himself to collect locusts surplus to requirements from a number of friends and provide them with a new home: the Palm House at Sefton Park. The parents of many of these friends were probably, like my mother, at their wits' end. They may not even have cared that the motives behind this apparent act of generosity leant more to mischief than altruism, but it was a divinely inspired mischief. His vision anticipated a link between modern biological science and the scriptures. Here was an opportunity to create a veritable plague of locusts.

Soon the word was out. Regular pilgrimages were being made to the scene of this unsanctioned experiment, even by pupils who had hitherto shown no interest in the natural world. Maybe they had been inspired by their divinity lessons. It wasn't long before an association was assumed by the staff at Sefton Park between the plague of schoolboys and the plague of locusts.

In truth the latter was putative. Perhaps the humidity was not congenial to locusts. Perhaps the place was saturated with organo-chlorides to suppress other pests. Perhaps the gardeners were alert and sprayed the strange invaders at the start. There were optimistic reports by some that 'there were hordes of them down there', but these budding journalists proved unreliable. When I visited there wasn't one to be seen, just the odd scowling staff member. We were never privy to what transpired in the corridors of power, but it would have been interesting to have been a locust on the wall.

'Due to a regrettable incident' the palm house was promptly declared out of bounds to boys in *our* school uniform.

~

Work makes heat. To demonstrate the Laws of Thermodynamics we repeatedly upended long cardboard tubes filled with small glass beads. After a while their temperature had risen measurably. Q.E.D. Later those same beads spirited from the lab were on the dining room floor, demonstrating the Laws of Motion. This experiment promised to be more diverting. A combination of properties contributed to the entertainment: a hard parquet floor, leather soled shoes (compulsory for all boarders), transparent invisibility and a sharp left turn into the dining area immediately through the doors. Add to this the desperate rush of those late boys keen to gain their seats before grace was said. Faces, full of intent and anxiety, were instantly transformed to surprise and alarm as centrifugal forces propelled them at a tangent to their intended destinations – a perplexing observation to all save a few mischief-makers. Perhaps the cleaners may have found a few small glass beads at the end of the day and wondered. For the rest of the diners it remained an unsolved mystery. For the miscreants it was good luck that no one was hurt. I admit to being irresponsible on occasion.

Mostly our pranks were innocuous enough. But if we could strike at the head of the system we would. Poor headmaster – at times we turned the tables on your power! If there was an 's' at the end of the line of that hymn, I can promise you that due accord was given to its sibilance: sonorously, slowly or almost silently – whisperingly, but always out of synchrony with our neighbours. These were the annoyances that all your threats of beatings and physical detentions were powerless to stop. Hold us back for extra hymn singing headmaster, if you must. The lessons we would miss were of more concern to you than us. See! You had to give up in defeat. The next day the sibilance was redoubled. Victory was ours. And when your dog pulled restlessly and disobediently on its lead at the school sports did you realise that you were entertaining a group of sixth-formers with a dog whistle? Being towed along by an eager Golden Retriever, your shooting-stick flailing, destroyed the image you affected. How interesting that dogs' hearing is far more sensitive than ours to sound of shorter wavelengths.

As figurehead of the whole rotten system, I felt little sympathy for you even when those irresponsible iconoclasts phoned every taxi firm in Liverpool on your behalf the day before the end-of-year break-up. They were timed to call round to your house at strategic intervals through the night, warned to knock at the door repeatedly because you were a little hard of hearing, and to please persist because you had a plane to catch. Was it my imagination that you looked tired as you shook my hand and wished me well on my journey through life? Nice sentiment, a shame you never knew my name.

Amid this curate's egg of a public school, the good parts succeeded in laying an education which would indeed propel me on life's journey. Over the decades I have retrospectively come to terms with the rest. Greater talents than mine have overcome far more serious hurdles. I may have had a privileged upbringing in the eyes of my erstwhile Taranaki colleague, Peter, and others who denounce English public schoolboys, but nothing is what it appears.

CHAPTER SIX

I WANTED TO BE A VET, BUT I NEVER HAD THE BRAINS

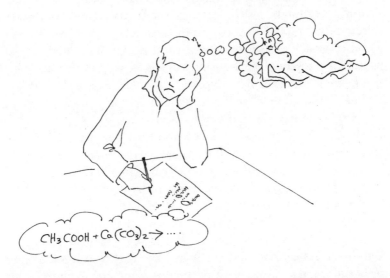

$$CH_3COOH + Ca(CO_3)_2 \rightarrow \cdots$$

I wanted to be a vet, but I never had the brains.' Most practising veterinarians would be able to dine out sumptuously and regularly if they were even moderately remunerated for the number of times they have had to field this statement, or its numerous variants, from their clients. Admittedly it is a declining refrain, and today's youth weaned on yuppie latte and Chardonnay marketing is more likely to iterate the disgusted 'yuk – the things some people have to do for a living'. We'll discuss the former sentiment first; the latter will become self-evident if you persist with this book.

Like many desirable things in life, attaining a difficult objective is a matter of luck, determination and ability. A deficiency in any one of these can be made up by a surfeit in another. I was certainly not regarded as a bright boy at school and the educational ethos of the day decreed that everyone should be made well aware of their deficiencies. School reports could be objects of dread. What parent would want to know that their child 'continues to know more and more, about less and less!'

Fortunately, in those days, the government fully funded tertiary education. However, five years' training for veterinarians was the most expensive of all degree courses for them to fund, and they wanted to make sure their investment was well targeted. From a national point of view, it made sense to try and ensure that a fair proportion of veterinary graduates ended up servicing the farming sector. Accordingly, most of the six veterinary schools in Britain selected their intake on the basis of interviews as well as 'A' level exam results. If you were from a rural background, had played rugby for the school 1st XV, and your neck was wider than your head, you could waltz in with three 'E' grades. If Barry Hardcastle had displayed his predilection for guinea pigs at such an interview, the bar would have been raised to three 'A's.

There was a very low intake of women. In my year there were forty students. Only seven of them were women and half of these had necks like water buffalo (I am relying on only three or four of them ever reading this ungracious fiction).

Nowadays selection from the thousands of applicants for the relatively few veterinary places is based solely on the seemingly fairer basis of academic ability. For many years the intake to veterinary colleges around the world has run at around seventy per cent women. Consequently there is a screaming shortage of rural veterinarians while the western world's pets have benefited immensely.

So how did I, Master Average, who never represented the school at rugby, had never been a prefect and only had a sixteen-inch collar, manage to be offered a place if I achieved three 'D's? It was all down to the interview.

First of all was the delicate matter of selecting to which of the six colleges to apply. I didn't really mind where, as long as I could be a vet at the end of it. My best chance would appear to be to apply to all six, but that would have been very naïve. These are unique and proud institutions. They would not understand how anyone could be promiscuous enough to want to achieve their degree anywhere without their own hallowed walls. Best to compromise and just apply to a maximum of three. There is always a hometown advantage, so in my case Liverpool had to be one of them. Their prospectus was enticing. It was set on glossy paper with black and white photos of eager students breezing about a modern campus in tweed jackets, collars and ties. This last gave away that the photos were, in fact, several years old; in the 1970s no self-respecting student would be seen in anything but denims and ponchos. For the more seriously left-wing, anti-establishment types, an expensive embroidered sheepskin jacket was *de rigueur* to show one's contempt for bourgeois, middle-class values. The buildings in this enticing brochure were also new looking, yet to be spoiled by the soot marks and other ravages that beset that ghastly sixties concrete and glass box architecture within months of erection. Liverpool wouldn't be too bad if I *had* to go there.

Of course really I wanted to be near the mountains. I had visions of weekends spent climbing and skiing in the Highlands, so my other applications were to Edinburgh and Glasgow. Edinburgh was a long shot. Their prospectus was written in gothic script on parchment and there were no pretty pictures. The Royal (Dick) [*sic*] College was obviously confident of its reputation and required no yuppy marketing (or the 1970s equivalent). What was more daunting to me was that half the prospectus appeared to be written in Latin and that inordinate emphasis seemed to be placed on accomplishment in this language. The introduction of Latin to our school syllabus had displaced Maths from the bottom of the division as far as my scholastic abilities were concerned, and Latin and Divinity were now my two weakest subjects at school. Any chance of this application succeeding was therefore a matter of faith, and consequently doomed to fail. I wasn't even granted an interview.

Glasgow, on the other hand, lured me into purchasing my first suit, and staying a risky night (redolent of Taggart) in the YMCA with some 'reformed' alcoholics, before rejecting me at interview. Although I was a desperately keen and passionate (though relatively untalented) cricketer, this cut no ice with one of the interviewers, who had obviously never heard of the game and only had ears for rugby. You could tell this because the ruckles on the inside of his had been smoothed out by repeated haematomas. Cauliflower ears are the hallmark of those who enjoy having them ground between the buttocks of their colleagues in this strange sport.

45

I currently work with both Glasgow and Royal (Dick) graduates and I can assure you that those colleges turn out a great product, although the Edinburgh graduates seem to have lapsed somewhat in the Classics of recent years.

Meanwhile, across the globe, aspiring colonials in New Zealand struggling merely to speak standard English (they will love me for this!) had to complete their veterinary education in Australian universities and further debase any linguistic skills they may have had. This undesirable state of affairs was reversed in 1968, the first year of intake for Massey University, when New Zealand started training its own vets. In New Zealand the requirements for university entrance are minimal, but there is a higher 'wastage' at the end of the first year of those who don't make the grade. This is perhaps a more equitable arrangement and should give late developers more chance. Alas for men! The end result is that in New Zealand, also, at least seventy per cent of those currently qualifying are women. They are, of course, graduates of the highest calibre and linguistically attuned to their unique and wonderful environment.

My suit purchase was not in vain. The interview at Liverpool hinged on an in-depth exploration of my knowledge of insectivorous plants, a topic I had listed as one of my interests on my application form. Fortunately I had (and still have) an abiding interest in plants of all types, but at that stage I was almost as well equipped to answer their questions as if they had asked me about mountain ranges round the world. The bar was set relatively low for me, but I didn't achieve my objective at first try.

The 'A' levels I required were Physics, Chemistry and Biology. It was Physics that I flunked. What was I to do? The prospect of another year at school was appalling. I had outgrown the system. I am now eternally grateful that my parents supported me for a year through Liverpool Polytech so that I could have another crack at my target. It wasn't going to be easy. At Polytech there were other distractions.

CHAPTER SEVEN

MUCH ADO ABOUT WOMEN

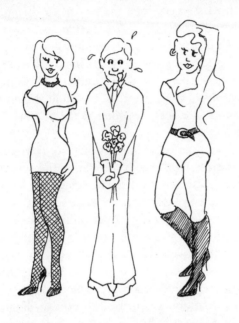

Lust is one of those glorious Anglo-Saxon words that has wandered from its Germanic origins. The original meaning yet lingers in the adjectival form. A *lusty* lad is one of vim and vigour; healthy and happy. Were he to be *lustful*, on the other hand, he would be prey to biblical sins. Physiologically lust is a primal driving force, essential to human survival, but it has the potential to disrupt social cohesion. One of the main determinants of cultural differences between different societies is how they harness this force and become, in their eyes, and often their eyes only, 'civilised'. The outward manifestations of a different culture may be subjected to derision – eating snails, men shaving armpits, as examples – but, deep down, the English envy the perceived sexual freedom of French society. Or did. Western, Anglo-Saxon dominated societies have changed vastly in the area of sexual mores since the end of the

Second World War, and the biggest changes seemed to coincide with my transition to manhood.

Adolescence is the period when an individual learns to adjust to the rules predetermined by the society or social group within which he/she lives. Successful adaptation depends on level of libido (difficult to control, even with cold showers) and strength of character (to break or obey the rules). Conscience plays the largest part. Middle-class English society used to be very efficient at implanting guilt complexes in its members – a torment unknown to the upper class and ignored by the uncivilised, lower classes. The balance of all these internal conflicts determines the thin veneer of civilisation that differentiates Englishmen from beasts of the field, and lesser societies such as the Spanish and, indeed, all other foreigners.

This transitional period is hard enough to navigate today, but for those of us growing through the sixties and seventies I would venture to say it was even harder. The rules were changing.

The first seventeen years of my life were spent almost entirely in the company of males, the only female influence being my mother. From the beginning her attitude towards the delicate subject of sexual morality borrowed heavily from her ancestors, a number of whom had been Methodist missionaries. Her father (the Professor) had a special interest in venereology, so her message of strict chastity was laced with pragmatism. To us the incoordinated steps of a drunkard weaving his way home along the pavement (a common sight in Liverpool) were not to be confused with the uncertain gait of those afflicted with *tabes dorsalis* (also a common sight in Liverpool), a terminal feature of untreated syphilis. The wages of sin were patently obvious. Spotting sinners was more fun than collecting number plates.

As children my brother and I were encouraged to read widely. At home we had a large selection of books from which to choose, and we absorbed a wide spectrum of literature, a lot of it dating from Edwardian times. I progressed from Beatrix Potter and The Brothers Grimm, to Rider Haggard, John Buchan and Robert Louis Stevenson. If mentioned at all, women in this genre of literature were to be revered. If they were beautiful they were invariably gentle and loving, and vice versa. Bad women were invariably ugly witches. Like all early childhood influences this was a hard one to dispel. I had imbibed an Edwardian attitude towards women and there were no role models to contradict it. We had no television.

As my fascination with the hidden world of women developed, I eagerly absorbed the eclectic works of J.B. Priestley, Howard Spring, Ernest Hemingway, Somerset Maugham, Guy de Maupassant and John Masters. The characters in their tales usually broke the rules of sexual etiquette: had affairs, committed adultery, or otherwise indulged in pre-marital or extra-marital sex. Those who broke the rules had the most fun and the most grief. Either way, it seemed they were the only ones worth writing about. No one ever got VD. If the principal characters married, sex between them was a taboo subject. End of novel. I have to declare that my interest was no longer pure: testosterone-laden fantasies tended to intrude. Biology dictated that I could no longer be true to my ideals. But would the well-honed guilt complex determine that I should never be free to indulge my secret longings?

I was often miserable in this 'unique' state, so close to ecstasy, so close to damnation. In the self-centred world of adolescence it didn't seem to register that ninety per cent of other young men also had spots and were in grave danger of going blind. If they were brought up in middle-class families they were mostly miserable, too. So woe to those men who tell you that school was the best time in their life. Either they were temporarily blessed (but in the long run cursed) with low libido or, more likely, they were about to embark on a career as a cad, unfettered by any taint of conscience. Ironically a high proportion of both sexes have always admired such men, witness society's infatuation with Hollywood and its denizens. Although the rules have changed (thank goodness), it is important to realise that there were always unwritten rules as well.

Liverpool Polytech was a melting pot for teenagers from all social backgrounds. Many of them would have arisen each morning from crusty sheets without a care in the world, and spoken to fair and fat alike without fear or favour. It would be a few years before I could aspire to that. At one level it was intoxicating. The presence even of Susan's hair clip on the next desk could evince paroxysms of longing, unrequited and destined to remain so. She was of course gorgeous, had a longstanding boyfriend, and to my enfeebled mind she was utterly unobtainable.

Ah Susan! That bright smile across the refectory table was
just for me.
I caught it and it seared my mind
An instant of blazing elation stabbed my heart
Yet I hung my head, unequal to your charming challenge,
Condemning myself to a year of agony
Inept, I tried to overcome that self-defeating lovelorn
gaucherie
And you were kind. That was so cruel!
Why did you forsake him for me that one weekend
And skilfully deflect my declaration ere it left my mouth?
I felt my heart would stop.
How different might our lives have been had I grasped the
moment?
And yet I know for me, a much wiser me,
That with you
I could never have been as happy as I have been.
Could our souls have truly soared when
Elvis hound-dogged through your mind,
But Elgar shook up me?

Losing the power of coherent speech in such circumstances is a major disadvantage. What would an experienced young lady want with a puppy like me? I contented myself with a flippancy that was quite well received and disguised my inner turmoil. Evidence of my desperation was manifest in my joining rehearsals for the production of *Trial by Jury*, just to be near her. I am not really a Gilbert and Sullivan fan and wild horses would not normally have induced me to contemplate setting one foot on a stage. Being cast as a 'little teapot' (short and stout) at primary school had been quite enough for me. It really didn't look as though anyone was ever going to be interested in me or my spout.

Yes, I had no idea how women's minds work (still don't, but then I have trouble with my own). However, despite such errors I knew that one day I would meet the love of my life, stop being a little animal and the pain would go away. All that literature had turned me into an incurable romantic. I now had a clear vision of what I wanted, not just for my career, but for my personal life. There was a lot to strive for.

The message is: if you have sons never, ever, send them to a single-sex school. In a modern, liberated society they will be at an almost insurmountable social disadvantage compared to those who have come from a co-educational background.

The major miracle was that I had survived my introduction to normal society still more or less sane and sat my three 'A' levels at the end of the year. I had several weeks to await the results.

CHAPTER EIGHT

NORWEGIAN INTERLUDE

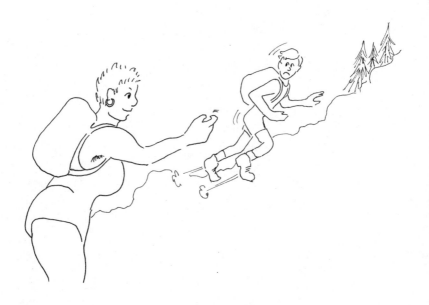

A couple of days after these exams John Watson and I were on a North Sea ferry. John, like me, had always had mountain fever and we arranged through a student agency to do voluntary work on farms in a remote part of Norway.

The Sognefjord is the longest fjord in Norway and slices deeply into its lonely mountains. Our anticipation grew as the boat slowly probed the calm waters from Balestrand, each twist in the Fjaerland arm revealing new vistas of rock and forest. From such isolated fastnesses fleets of Viking longboats had carried fierce men seawards in the Dark Ages to plunder, ravage and ultimately settle softer lands across the North Sea. Their feats of seamanship, their courage, and the fear generated by their berserk blood-lust changed the course of European history.

It seemed strange to contrast these images with the sun-dappled peace of the glistening fjord that John and I surveyed. The bows gently parted the hissing water, and the deck strummed beneath our feet. Cadences of Edvard Grieg surged and echoed in my mind. Great was our excitement as we disembarked down the small wooden gangway, well and truly freed from our city-centred lives.

Fjaerland, a small farming and tourist community, nestled at the head of a northern branch of the Sognefjord. Two glaciers descended almost to sea level through breaches in the mountain rampart which held back the vast Jostedal ice-cap. Between them their retreat had left a pocket-handkerchief of fertile soil, providing the toe-hold on which these Viking descendants survived. In 1968 it was only accessible by boat – the way we had come. We revelled in our good fortune to have chosen such a magic spot. It was picture postcard perfect.

In such regions farmers' livestock has to be wintered indoors for seven months of the year, a major disadvantage compared with Britain (three to five months), or New Zealand where it is possible to dispense with the major cost of wintering accommodation altogether. The old wooden house where I was hosted took advantage of hot air rising, and the cattle were housed under the living quarters during winter. However, John and I were here for the summer, a time of frenetic activity when seven months' worth of hay and silage has to be made in the space of a few weeks of rather dubious weather. Norwegian farmers are grateful for all the help they can get over this period and eager foreign students looking for adventure readily fit the bill. Luck was to be with us this year; it turned out to be one of the driest summers on record.

My host farmer, Ivar, took me to my first task. A large field with rows of turnips awaited my inexperienced ministrations. I was given a hoe, shown what was required, and left to my own devices. It was raining. Within an hour or so my hands were blistering and I wondered how I would last two months. Peer Gynt was starting to become repetitive. Even the best meals can cause indigestion.

It was not as though I had received a warm welcome. The family seemed dysfunctional in some way; a late marriage with one incredibly spoilt young son. Ivar was always fair to me, if rather distant, and chose to use his reasonable English very sparsely. Communication was problematical, especially at the start. I slept in an outhouse and wasn't included in family life. The suit I had been told to bring, because social life in Norway 'is very formal', hung forlornly on a nail in my damp room against the peeling wallpaper for my whole stay. Dust from the woodworm snowed onto its shoulders.

None of this seriously troubled me because I was entranced by my surroundings. I could set aside that hoe and look at the vast sweeping rock face of Blånipa (Blue Peak) across the valley. 5000 feet above me his misty head parted the mantle of the icecap. I still recall the best photograph I have never taken when one late, balmy afternoon I was descending from a walk high above the valley, where I had been visiting a sirtah (a summer hut providing access to the high meadows). As I rounded a bend in the track, admiring the light streaming round the shoulders of Blånipa, a woman with a wooden yoke across her shoulders and two pails walked out of history and into the foreground. That moment was for me one of heart-stopping sublimity.

When I had recovered from my heart attack I resumed my merry way.

After the hoeing, silage and haymaking started in earnest. In this wet climate haymaking was very labour intensive. When the cut grass had wilted it was hung on specially constructed fences and, once dry, the loose hay was manhandled into a horse-drawn cart and unloaded into a large barn with slat sides. For silage a tower was constructed from spars arranged in a circle and wired together. Johan, a local lad, used a buck rake on the back of the tractor to sweep cut grass towards this structure. The real workers, arranged at the base of the tower, tossed forkfuls of this onto the growing heap within. After several weeks of alternately pitching the grass into the tower and trampling it down, and pulling grass and hay on and off fences, I started coveting his job.

Never mind, I was getting lean and fit on this hard work and a rather meagre diet (just wait till Ivar junior became a ravenous teenager) comprising largely goats' milk cheese, tough stew and fruit soup. But, damn it, Johan was glued to that tractor seat and seemed decidedly reluctant to spill any of *his* gravy. Ivar must have noticed this and I was promised that one day I, too, could drive the tractor. Eventually that day arrived and Gunar, an older farm worker, who had been coming to the farm for many years – a kind man of peasant disposition – stepped onto the buck rake behind me. *He* had never been allowed to drive the tractor. Off I drove down the road towards the bridge. As we approached it Gunar seemed to be saying something to me. Was it exhilaration that caused the increased animation in his voice? I throttled onto the narrow wooden bridge. It was quite bumpy. Bump, bump, bump. Strange, when the road surface was smooth. Another thing: although Gunar's voice seemed to be louder, it was yet more distant.

Gunar had done the wise thing and jumped off before the buck rake (which was wider than the tractor – silly me not to have noticed) had demolished the handrail and supporting struts one by one. This was one bridge that wasn't likely to help the gap between cultures. To his credit Ivar was very restrained, but I wouldn't describe him as being best pleased. I pulled my head in and worked harder than ever after that, but for some reason I was never allowed near the tractor again. In the end I must have redeemed myself. I noted in my diary when I was preparing to leave that Ivar said, 'You must go back so early? You can stay here as long as you like. We are so very satisfied!'

John's farm was adjacent to one of the glaciers and his host, Anders, was a far more convivial personality. Anders was the proud possessor of an alpine hut set on a ridge 3000 feet above the valley floor. In return for ferrying supplies, such as the odd bag of cement (he certainly made use of us as we got fitter), we were allowed free rein up there. From this magnificent eyrie it was possible to don skis and set out across the Jostedal icecap. On many a weekend we would carry supplies up for Anders and cross-country ski or borrow a tent and camp out on the rocky nunataks – islands in a sea of snow and ice. Vast panoramas unrolled. Away to the east were the Jotunheim, home to the frost and rock giants of Norse mythology, and Norway's highest peaks. The silence and isolation were magical. Nearby, delicate alpine plants survived in the sun-warmed fissures of the rock. Sometimes we were accompanied by other students on these trips, usually Danish or Norwegian, who also worked on Anders' farm. This was a relief, because they invariably spoke good English and were able to show us the ropes and inform us about the area.

One weekend, Brita and Ingrid, two Norwegian university students, joined us. It was a hot sunny day as Anders loaded us with extra provisions for his hut. A summer of physical work had hardened us well to the task and we steadily pulled up the steep climb from the valley floor despite our heavy packs. John and Ingrid were ahead. I was last: following behind Brita's pumping legs. These Norwegian girls were fit. As the track levelled off she turned round.

'Look, John, I will show you something.'

Her English, as usual, was perfect. She beckoned me off the track to a small declivity. Dotting the short-cropped grasses were alpine flowers. Some I recognised from British hills – Milkwort and Parsley fern – but many, like the neat little four-petalled Cornel, were new and exotic to me. Below we could see the track we had climbed and across to the fjord and its jumble of surrounding peaks. Brita dropped her pack and sat on the sweet grass in the hollow. I joined her. It was cool relief to lose that weight and feel my sweat-soaked shirt separate from the skin of my back.

'Maybe we should take off some clothes.'

Had I heard correctly?

'It's hot, John, we should take off our clothes. The others won't mind if we're a little late.'

Yes, there was no mistaking this. I had a strong notion that if I complied with the suggestion there would be consequences for which I was totally unprepared. Brita was a strapping specimen of Norse womanhood. I liked her, but I didn't fancy her in the least. I had followed those sturdy suntanned legs uphill for a couple of hours without a tinge of lust. I think it was the crew-cut. What really surprised me was that there had been no sign of tenderness on her part. No evidence that I was a favoured one. She had told us about her boyfriend in Bergen and how he was soon to come and join her. Perhaps I had misunderstood – nakedness has less significance for Nordic races than the average Brit – but her disappointed, even scornful, response to my gabbled excuses as I grabbed my pack left me doubting. Had I refused an offer that no red-blooded male ever should, or had she read my misunderstanding and was outraged at my presumption? Was I in her eyes a gauche mouse, or an arrogant male? Neither was a wholesome option.

Literature is filled with heroes who have known how to react in such situations. We all know what Flashman (at least in George MacDonald Fraser's re-incarnation) would have done. I wondered about Tom Brown. He would have done the manly thing, graciously. What was that? As a callow, nineteen-year-old I had no idea. I didn't know the rules in my own country, let alone these strange shores. Yet scorn has an international language, and Brita needed no great skill to stab me with her over-powering disdain. As we walked on to the hut it was as though a cloud had come over the sun and the blooms had lost their charm. Not for the first or last time in my life, I was in the throes of self-doubt. I had a lot of thinking to do.

If this had been an opportunity to lose my virginity I couldn't have chosen a better setting, but my upbringing had prepared me for a spiritual experience with someone I loved, preferably a woman suffused with pre-Raphaelite beauty. A quick shag with the mannish Brita didn't quite fit the bill. We can't discard the values instilled in us at the drop of a hat. I had been steeped in the 'middle-class ethic of postponed pleasure'. This applied as much to sex, as to saving the choicest roast potato on my plate till last, or delaying unwrapping the Christmas presents till late morning. *All good things come to he who waits.* Women who claim that men are only after one thing misunderstand. Chivalry, chemistry and due courtship are requisite precursors for many of us. I consoled myself that although I had been a mouse on this occasion, a spiritual man was within me.

Society moves on, but I still hold to my own inclination – that chastity is a virtue to be broken *only in good taste*. This seemingly bold statement is as open to interpretation as any biblical injunction. It is a guiding principle to which I have vehemently adhered: a rule of which Tom Brown, and even Flashman *were he the judge*, would have approved.

The after-effects of this awkward weekend stretched to months and years, but I finally made sense of them yesterday.

~

One of the least useful things that I had brought with me, along with my suit, was a *Teach Yourself Norwegian* book. The contents bore little resemblance to what my ears were telling me. However, after two months with its limited help I was very proud that I could make myself at least partially understood. What I didn't realise was that I had picked up a dialect of Landsmål, a tongue of the Western seaboard and more akin to the language of the Vikings than the main Riksmål language, which more closely resembles Danish. When we returned home via Bergen, people failed to understand even my basic 'yes' and 'no'. I had to admit defeat and resort to the shame of most English people abroad: using my native tongue.

It was a combination of technical failure and linguistic incompatibility that led to an incident of incredible frustration for me towards the end of my stay. While I had been sampling an idyll some unfortunate desk-bound academics were slaving away back in England marking my 'A' level efforts. My whole future rested on these exam results, but this wonderful sojourn had allowed me to put the burning issue of my future career to the back of my mind. Suddenly, one day, I was summoned by Ivar to the phone. On the end of the line I could hear my mother's voice chatting to my father as she waited for a connection.

'It will be interesting to hear how he reacts when he hears the news...'

'Hello, Mummy, can you hear me?'

'... especially when he wasn't expecting to know until he came back... Come on, blast you! Why can't we get through?'

My mother is not the most patient of people, especially in situations like this.

'Mummy, I'm here. I can hear you perfectly. Please, please just tell me the results!'

'Dors was gobsmacked when she heard. She had no idea that he would get anywhere near.'

Me, exasperatedly (I share my mother's genes), 'For God's sake, just spout out the bleeding results!'

My mother, seeking to cast blame, 'We can't get through, we can't get through. Some silly swine can't have pressed the right switch at the other end.'

Operator, to me, in perfect English, 'I'm very sorry, sir, but it is not possible to make a connection.'

'But can you hear her?'

'Yes, sir.'

'Well, please could you just ask her to state my exam results over the line. I can hear every word she's saying perfectly. They are very important to me.'

'I regret that there is another operator and she can't understand.'

Click, click. Followed a little later by, 'I'm very sorry, sir, but she's hung up.'

For a brief uncharitable moment that's precisely what I wanted to do to my dearest mother.

It was to be another ten days before that tantalising hint was verified. I felt such relief and joy. Despite the best efforts of testosterone I had the grades and was soon to start my first year at Liverpool University Veterinary Faculty.

CHAPTER NINE

TEASERS AND PIZZLES

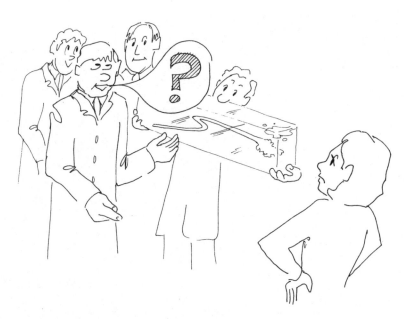

pizzle (´pizəl) n., (archaic or dialect), the penis of an animal, esp. a bull [ETYMOLOGY 1523, from L.Ger. pesel or Flem. pezel, dim. of root of Du. pees 'sinew', from O.L.G. root*pisa. Alternatively, and less prissily (JH) resulting from elision of 'piss' O.F. pissier urinate, and 'hole'.]

Mae Coster was one of us. One of a small group of forty new 'fresher' veterinary students about to be put through the humiliation of an initiation ceremony at the hands of older and supposedly more worldly-wise veterinary students. She was the one selected from our group to go to the front of the lecture theatre and identify the formalinised specimen that had been smuggled down from the anatomy laboratory. It was, as she rightly and disdainfully declared, a bull's penis. She gave the impression that she had a vast experience of all types of penis and that this one did not particularly impress her, an attitude that took her questioner aback.

Perhaps a few years earlier a blushing new graduate would have provided entertainment for those assembled, but those days had gone. The rules had changed. The meeting ended in anticlimax.

Mae's attitude was at one level surprising. The specimen would have been almost a metre long if fully extended. But Mae was the product of a co-educational system and who knows what might have been lurking behind the bike sheds in Wolverhampton? I was frightened off her immediately.

When I started working in rural New Zealand I occasionally encountered bulls with injured penises. A bull's penis is in fact a rigid fibrous organ and erection is achieved mostly by muscular contraction straightening out an 'S' bend. If the protruded penis is not on target for intromission it is possible for penile tissue to rupture and block off the urethra. Unable to urinate, such a bull will slowly die without veterinary intervention. On large farms, where cattle are not checked every day, the problem may not be apparent till the accumulation of urine under the skin of the belly is noticed, a condition called 'water belly'. By this stage the bull will be looking decidedly seedy. Since surgery to restore full working capability is expensive and generally unsuccessful, the usual procedure is to create an opening in the urethra under the anus so that urine flow is restored, albeit in an unusual direction for a bull. The surgery is done with the bull standing, using an epidural anaesthetic to deaden pain. In advanced cases there is often rotten tissue in the vicinity from urine leakage, in which case penis amputation is required. Withdrawing a metre-long bull's penis from a small incision under the bull's tail is one of the more dramatic moments in veterinary surgery.

The farmer is left with a bull which it is dangerous to stand behind when not wearing wet-weather gear, and a defunct penis. The latter is discarded or scavenged by the farm dog. The bull may recover to be salvaged for meat (probably hamburgers), or (the bull's preference) retained as a 'teaser' to select cows on heat for artificial insemination.

Teasers were widely used until it was discovered that other cows are better at detecting when their friends have 'come on' and all that is needed is to put some paint on the cows' backs and see when it gets rubbed off. Vasectomies were not the method of choice for making a bull infertile and turning him into a teaser, because in theory the bull could still, in his promiscuous perambulations, spread venereal diseases; a consideration that is frequently lacking in the human model. One ingenious solution was an operation to alter the angle of the bull's penis by a few degrees so that he was unable to insert and fired blanks to one side. Bovine lovemaking is singularly unimaginative and, without recourse to the Kama Sutra, such a bull was condemned to an unsatisfying sex-life. The success of this method relied on the long time it took before reason over-ruled instinct and the bull realised that there was no reward for the effort and gave up in disgust.

The penis? One of my colleagues had a use for that, and on one occasion had requested that I save it. I duly put it in a plastic bag when the farm dog wasn't looking and concealed it in my car.

Sean is a likeable Irishman with a great sense of humour, and hanging a penis from the rafters of your garage is eccentric behaviour beyond the bounds required to claim affiliation with even this noble race. But there was method in his madness.

At her birthday party a very attractive and worldly lady with a passion for horses was presented with a long, slender, and elegantly wrapped package containing the by now well-dried and decidedly whippy article. Bull pizzles are apparently used in other parts of the world as riding crops. She carried the moment with as much panache as Mae had a few years earlier. The end product was an aesthetic disaster, but extremely serviceable; a possible accessory for rodeo, but definitely not for the refined dressage circles to which this lady aspired.

CHAPTER TEN

ANATOMY OF A VETERINARY STUDENT

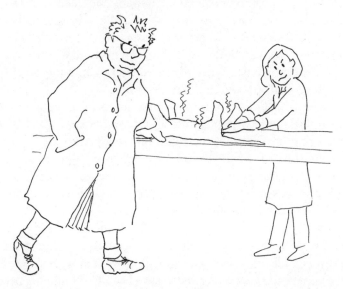

The anatomy library housed many more spectacular specimens. Heavy, formalin-filled Perspex boxes glugged as avid students tilted them for close inspection. On surreal shroud-white flesh snaked lurid blood vessels, injected with coloured resin. Diaphanous veils of tissue wafted on unseen currents, snowstorms of scurfy debris swirled. There is no refuge; there are no secrets in this pellucid prison: all is revealed by the anatomist's scalpel. Is this all science? Is there no room for awe? Who can gaze on such relics without some passing thoughts on their own mortality? Or reflect on the sometimes sordid history of the early men of learning whose curiosity about the body drove them to such an unnatural pursuit?

Ah! Here is the delicate dissection of an eye of newt.

Be careful! Do not shake me,
For the williwaws of detritus you create
Will but haste the ravages of time, and speed my final fate.

And so, in the main, these relics are accorded the respect they deserve.

Barry Hardcastle struggled for a mnemonic, something that would help him to remember the sequence of nerves conjoining at the brachial plexus: something suitably obscene. He was ably assisted by others. Soon we had created a phrase replete with sexual connotations that would never bear repeating in polite company, but memorable long after we had forgotten the assignations of the initial letters. We were juveniles adjusting to an adult world; you must forgive us the odd lapse in decorum.

Those who had joined the course lured by images of caring individuals tenderly bandaging dogs' paws, or some bucolic idyll, were being re-educated, their illusions stripped to the bone. This was the start of a five-year science degree. Subjects that seemed remote from our ultimate objective – in nearly all cases to become a practising vet – were drummed into us. Organic chemistry, biochemistry, physiology: all were subjects with which I struggled and even, one stressful summer, had to re-sit. The dread of having to repeat a year was sufficient spur for me to pass but, for me, a pass was a pass and that was enough. I wanted to be a vet. I was never going to be honours material. Honours graduates perform consistently highly throughout the full five years of the course. Perhaps only one student in forty would attain this standard. I held on to my rustic dreams.

Later studies such as pharmacology, microbiology and genetics built on those early courses and by the time we entered our third year it was possible to see an end to academia. We would soon be bandaging dogs' paws, but we would know the underlying principles of pathology and pharmacology that govern healing and therapy. We would soon be leaning on that sunny gate beside the farmer, discussing the state of his stock, but with some knowledge of ruminant physiology, animal husbandry and nutrition.

Our studies were intensive, a stream of lectures filled our days. We were effectively separated from other more social students studying non-vocational subjects. Some of the social science students had only two or three lectures a week, for goodness' sake! They could indulge their individual voyages of self-discovery and uphold the student stereotype of political protest and free love, and fulfil peacenik ideals whilst collecting money for the IRA. Our lot was different, more a matter of endurance, application and enquiry. There was very little free time for a plodder like me. As the course progressed and became more practical and shed its Perspex perspective, it became more enjoyable, but I would never contend, as some do, that university years were the best of my life. They were years of unremitting study.

I was also assailed by doubts as to where my vocation would lead. Field trips to farms nearby in Cheshire to familiarise us with modern production systems were far from my experience and conception of what rural life should involve. Pigs reared in sweatboxes and other intensive pig and poultry systems alarmed me. This trend to factory farming even extended to dairy cows housed under zero-grazing systems, where the grass was cut and brought to them. As we wandered around screeching pig factories it was obvious that my disillusionment was shared by other students, in part because the noise, dust and smell made it a far from ideal learning environment. Peter Piggott, however, seemed indifferent to this and was enjoying the status of his new waders.

Many British vets in those days wore fishermen's waders because they frequently had to work with housed cattle on deep litter systems. Because straw is added to the accumulating dung the vet called in to examine a sick animal may be walking on a thick layer of dung and straw. If the farmer has been mean with the straw the vet will be walking *in* thick slurry. For farm vets a pair of thigh-length waders and a brown coat were desirable accoutrements.

Peter had acquired his shiny new waders a trifle early in our estimation. He was getting ideas above his station for a second-year student; although his swaggering gait may have been misinterpreted. Traipsing around for an hour or so on a summer's day in waders full of pig nuts, posted unobligingly by friends and colleagues, made the swagger at first obligatory: later a stagger. Even a stylish individual would not find it easy to pull off waders and empty them of pig food in the middle of acres of slurry, with any degree of élan. In fact it is not an everyday conundrum and to our disappointment it presented a challenge that Peter was disinclined to meet. He was a hulking and clumsy youth, but he had dignity, and he defused our mirth by ignoring our childish antics; we learned the more because of it. We were growing up. No one else ever wore waders.

It was difficult to adjust to the freer and more collaborative relationships that we had with our university lecturers. For my part, strict schooling had precluded any social interaction between teachers and pupils. Teachers like 'Mong' (of whom we shall hear more) kept an icy remove from their students. Schoolboys must be kept in line, any glimmer of weakness and life as a master would be intolerable: them or us.

For students at university by contrast, it was a matter of self-motivation. The lecturers were a diverse bunch. For many of them teaching was a minor aside to their research. If their teaching was lame or inadequate it was up to us to do the background reading and make good the deficits in our knowledge or understanding. No one was going to write a sardonic report to your parents if you were performing inadequately.

Students of brilliance were able to transcend the boundaries and freely discourse with these higher mortals, but those treading the fine line between pass and fail, such as me, were acutely aware of the sway they held. They still marked those exam papers. Your future was in their hands and some of them consciously wielded this power.

Miss Jericho bestrode the pathology lab in ankle socks and plimsolls, her rotund figure concealed under a long white coat, her short grey hair worn in a pragmatic manner that owed nothing to elegance. She was about to show who was boss in a rather unusual manner.

The dead dogs lay coldly on the tables: strays that had been euthanased and arranged for us to venture on our first tentative forays into the intricacies of surgery. A moment of eager anticipation was tempered fractionally by the cloying stench of death. But before we began, Miss Jericho wanted to involve us in a particular interest of hers. Dog pox...

'The lesions are barely detectable. They are occasionally visible on the mucosa of the prepuce in the male dog, as with this dog that Miss Coster is examining. Far more difficult to detect are the lesions in the rectal mucosa. You will need to palpate carefully and for this purpose you may not use a finger cot because it reduces tactile

66

sensitivity too much. I repeat: these lesions are barely detectable. You must use a naked finger. If any of you find any lesions, please let me know. There is plenty of disinfectant and there are brushes by the basin at the right.'

And so I present, for your delectation, an unusual vignette. Forty students put to an exacting test. How will they perform in the brown finger stakes? Some caught in the enthusiasm of the moment dived in with nary a thought. For others, years of civilised conditioning was waging a winning battle with their scientific inquisitiveness. This was Miss Jericho's real experiment. None of us would hear about 'dog pox' ever again. Her beady eyes, glinting over the steel half-frame spectacles, spotted a malingerer.

'Well, Mister Hardcastle, have you checked to see if your dog has rectal lesions?'

'Not yet, Miss Jericho, I'm just about to.'

And so, right there and then and under the direct supervision of the expert, he performed the manipulation to her satisfaction. Sometimes it is better to feign enthusiasm and lie.

'Has this dog got dog pox, Mister Hicks?'

'No, Miss Jericho.' (I decided to rely on the laws of probability.)

'Let me check... No, your dog seems to be clear.' (And for once they were on my side.)

I always seemed to get on reasonably well with Miss Jericho after that. She was my exacting tutor in the final clinical year.

Most other lecturers were more innocuous. If anybody fitted the role of the absent-minded professor more completely than 'Piggy' I have yet to meet them. Piggy was our animal husbandry lecturer, and yes, he did have an interest in pigs, but that was not the sole reason for his nickname. Piggy was just a remarkably bumbling and untidy figure. His florid complexion was curtained by lank, greying locks. His tweed jacket was invariably strung up to the wrong button. When Piggy farted home it was in a car not seen in present times, in fact a rare beast even then. Piggy owned the only Wartburg on the campus. A car attuned to his needs. This wasn't the saloon version. This was a Wartburg estate: ideal for the discerning pig farmer. You could hump all the pails of swill you required into its roomy abdomen. A car as un-dashing and inelegant as its name implies.

Another professor, on the other hand, drove a Rover. He was ever dapper, and invariably sported a blazer and bow tie. His lectures were accomplished, amusing and opinionated, but his politics were conservative and he deplored the bohemian appearance of many of the students. He was not amused by the 'Vote Labour' sticker that one wag affixed to the rear window of his car while he was having drinks at his club. He was especially mortified that several days elapsed before it was brought to his attention.

Slowly but surely, inappropriate thinking was eliminated from our repertoire. Physiology was my intellectual bête noire. The standards expected were laid from the beginning.

'I shall expect no student to revert to *this*,' said the professor of physiology, disdainfully displaying a copy of Greene. Greene was an excellent little text that in simple terms gave an overview of a complex topic. 'This is Noddy physiology.'

I had never been an Enid Blyton fan and dismissing Noddy came naturally to me, but this time it was a big mistake – I didn't discover the virtues of Greene until I was in the process of re-sitting my physiology paper. And so we were directed to my nemesis, the dense and frightening tome of Stirling: over a thousand pages of angstrom units and other worthy physiological esoterica that seemed more designed to obfuscate than enlighten.

But even a dry topic can be leavened by the inspired eccentricities of a great mind. The cardinal sin was teleology. Teleology is the mistake of confusing, for instance, anatomical design in terms of purpose. A giraffe doesn't have a long neck *so* that it can feed off high branches, but *because* having a long neck has given it an evolutionary advantage, enabling it to feed off high branches that other animals cannot reach. Lamark versus Darwin. To illustrate the point the professor was fond of resorting to an obscure avian example.

'The Red Vented Bulbul...' a name he enunciated elaborately, lovingly caressing each syllable, '...ladies and gentlemen, with which I am sure by now all of you have more than passing familiarity, is so named because it has a red vent. It does not have a red vent because it is called the Red Vented Bulbul'.

Idiosyncrasies aside, our lecturers were for the most part role models of scientific excellence and integrity, determined to cast intellectual shoddiness from their charges; men and women to whom we could look up and hope to emulate in a lifelong pursuit of logic and objectivity.

~

'Daddy, why don't you ever read us *The Tale of Little Red Riding Hood*?'

'I can't, darling; I just don't enjoy it any more. When I was your age I loved it, but my tertiary education has made me aware that it was full of the crassest teleological thinking.'

'Oh, do try, Daddy. The wolf was just ignorant. He didn't know that it was eons of evolution that had given him such big eyes, big teeth and big ears. If Little Red Riding Hood had tried to correct his teleological explanations he would have got very, very angry.'

CHAPTER ELEVEN

STUDENT IN THE DALES

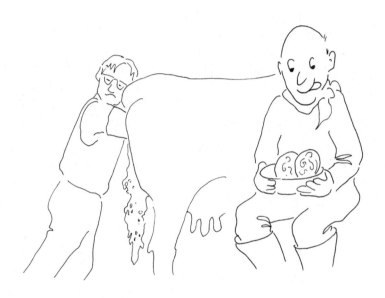

Meanwhile my faith in my future in the profession was restored each holiday as I saw practice with a remarkable vet based in the Yorkshire Dales, an area to which my parents had moved. Here there was no intensive agriculture, but a pattern of sweeping fells, stone walls, forested gills and flag-roofed barns. It was more than picturesque. This was and, thanks to the National Park status that it enjoys, still is a beautiful corner of England, but facilities were primitive. Mike's predecessor was a retired army officer who had trundled around his patch with a horse and trap. Mike had modernised and over several years we patrolled the twisty lanes in a succession of Landrovers.

This was stiff-shit country and Mike never wore waders, but he did wear a brown coat. A brown coat without waders or water-proof over-trousers is an impractical combination, the nature of the work leading inevitably to brown knees. Even today it seems requisite, in British veterinary journal advertisements put out by drug companies, to depict vets in brown coats. New Zealand vets, clad in practical green overalls, may wonder the reason for this, but it is quite simple. It is a matter of professional image. An 'overall' in Britain is often referred to as a 'boiler suit' and therefore worn by labourers. We can't have that, can we?

Mike faced the world in a brown tweed jacket, brown trousers and always wore a collar and tie. On entering a barn full of rollicking calves the jacket would come off, to be hung in some cobwebbed corner. If it was a big job the tie might join it. I would be given the task of bulldogging the calves if there was insufficient labour (clasping them round the neck with one arm whilst gripping the septum of the nose firmly between the thumb and index finger of my other hand to restrain them), while Mike went down on his knees (now browner and wetter) and castrated them. On the odd farm the farmer might doff his cloth cap and Mike would place the steaming hot testicles within. What culinary delight was conjured up from such an unpromising start I know not, but the practice was guaranteed to result in a sticky head and, only if you were lucky, a hairy chest.

So we went, from farm to farm. You have read all about it in the wonderful series of books written by James Herriot. For people around the world the physical beauty of the countryside in which I was privileged to get an early grounding as a vet has been made accessible by the television series based on those books.

As we journeyed I was encouraged to reflect and question what we had done, what we might have done and, occasionally, what we should have done. A chance to glean a lifetime's experience is rare indeed and I like to think that he enjoyed my company. In return I opened many gates for him.

Mike had firm ideas about most things. It was manly to ignore discomfort; indeed discomfort was a part of the job. My hands froze as I recorded while he TB-tested Galloway cattle up on the fells in the cruel frosts of winter. We returned damp and dirty to his Landrover after blood-testing handfuls of cattle housed in barns scattered across the fields. Walking was often the only means of access, sometimes in drenching rain. We treated wretched, scouring calves lying in the stinking ordure of their bracken bedding, and we rolled in slimy shippons to calve cows. Life behind that bucolic façade was often hard and brutal. The lack of facilities for handling animals, such as races and head-bails, made the job frustratingly inefficient and occasionally dangerous. How ironic then, that Mike should have succumbed to an unseen invader.

Mike firmly believed that a healthy and vigorous life kept the bugs at bay. He disdained the use of many conveniences that would now be regarded as essential. One of the worst tasks facing vets is removing retained placentas from cows. In the normal course of events a cow will naturally eject her placenta within a few hours of birth. Occasionally the placental attachments to the uterus will not part and the placenta is retained within the cow, usually leaving a smelly wick of rapidly rotting tissue dangling by the tail. Farmers are not best pleased by this state of affairs because placing the cups of the milking machine on the udder beside that swishing tail can defeat the subsequent efforts of even the best after-shave lotion (make that scrubbing brush and carbolic soap – we are talking of Yorkshiremen here after all). The temptation is to intervene as soon as possible. Nowadays, research has shown that the best approach is to remove any protruding membranes and allow natural dehiscence, only intervening if the cow is sick. Until this divine statistical analysis of outcomes was widely published vets were routinely called out if the cow hadn't 'cleansed' within four days. This meant the tedious task of trying to unbutton numerous placental attachments, all the while causing collateral damage that could result in infertility, but at least the cow didn't stink any more and milking her became more pleasant.

Long-sleeved plastic gloves protect the hands and arms of the operator from the hot bacterial soup within the uterus and help ensure that he/she will be welcomed home, if not with open arms, at least with only mild repudiation. Unfortunately one of the commonest reasons for retained membranes is because the cow has aborted and, until the disease was eradicated later in the last century, one of the commonest causes of abortion was *Brucella abortus*. This bacterium has been the death of many vets and farmers.

Mike maintained that wearing gloves impaired the sensitivity of the fingers required to separate the rotting placenta from the uterus. He wore gloves because he got a rash on his arms if he didn't, but he compromised their protective effect by cutting off the fingertips. Even had he left them intact, he would still have been at risk. Gloves were often defective and tore or gave way at the seams. A healthy constitution is no defence against brucellosis, and it is a condition difficult to diagnose in humans because of its range of manifestations. It is truly debilitating and not easily treated, even with modern antibiotics. After initial symptoms that can be mistaken for flu it may become chronic, cause heart problems, settle into joints and even result in neurological and psychological changes.

Mike and his wife lived in a large stone house with cobbled drive. Inside, the polished oak panelling and parquet floor gleamed. We always had time for lunch and it was always something substantial, even exotic – grouse, pheasant, trout. His wife was a wonderful cook. This was style and Mike, notwithstanding those stained trouser knees, had it in oodles. He had been the sole vet in a remote area for years. He had been on duty night and day to service the needs of a demanding clientele – not that the dour Yorkshire farmers would appreciate such a fancy foreign appellation. He was widely respected in the community and his loss to brucellosis, perhaps ten years later, was keenly felt.

For me, the doubts remained. I didn't think the glory was worth the discomfort. I belonged to a softer generation.

CHAPTER TWELVE

AND THEN THERE WAS YOU

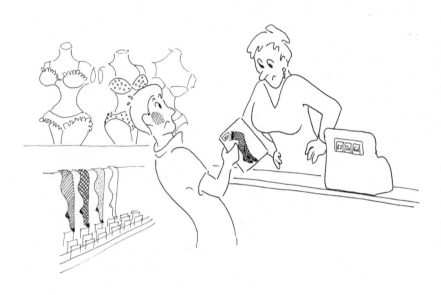

Once upon a time, two soldiers of misfortune manned the guns that defended the great city of London from the worst that Hitler could fling at it. Their misfortune was that their birthdates decreed that they would be embroiled, along with millions of others, in the cataclysmic upheaval that was the Second World War. One was my father, ex-public school. His passions were motor cycling, gliding, the great outdoors. He stood to inherit the family bakery business, but his ability in maths initially suggested a more academic career. The war was to change that. The other, the son of a builder, had spent his formative years during the Great Depression in a damp and claustrophobic mining town in South Wales. He had left school at fourteen, left his father's employ a few years later and was a pantry boy at a public school when war broke out. Despite any disadvantages of upbringing, he is a man of spirit, a natural comedian who can wring laughter from a basset hound.

My fortune was that war forged an enduring friendship between these two men. During the war my father was best man at the wedding of his friend and subsequently the annual Christmas card was for many years the tenuous link between them and their growing families.

When I was in my early teens the families met briefly as the Lanfears passed through Liverpool on their way to a holiday in Scotland. The youngest daughter was a gorgeous little blond thing. Little did I know how she was to blossom.

Our next encounter was during another family visit several years later. I had just finished my first year at university, with the ignominy of an organic chemistry re-sit exam hanging over me. Here was an attractive, charming girl: natural and kind. A Frenchman, to my chagrin (what else), had once described her as 'sympathique', and though I regarded him as competition at the time, I concede it is entirely fitting.

I have it on reliable authority that the feeling was mutual. How was I to know that? I touched her arm and it was not withdrawn, was there even a reassuring little squeeze in return? Further opportunities for less ambiguous displays of affection did not arise within the confines of a family visit. I have touched many arms before and since, but this was the memorable one, the one that quickened heart, mind and soul; yet it was meaningless if it had no significance to its recipient.

Women are much better at this sort of thing than men. Their intuitive skills enable them to move with assurance through the shadowy, blurred and insubstantial world of love and emotion. To those males of more Neanderthal persuasions there is no hindrance; you see the apple and you pluck it. Some apples (Brita?) like to be plucked. Why go through all the angst? Civilisation has complicated the rules of the game. It decrees that the apple shall not be plucked by a civilised man unless it wants to be and that if the picker has been to an English public school he shall have both hands tied behind his back. If he is a Neanderthal who happens to have gone to an English public school he will pretend to have his hands tied. All the while that little apple can decide whether to drop into his mouth or dok him on the head, or pretend to do either. It knows whether he is there just for a casual nibble or to satisfy a lifelong craving. All power to the apple; who would have it otherwise? Men may as well have their feelings tattooed on their foreheads for all their body language and chemistry reveals to the fairer sex. Men require more tangible proofs of affection and commitment.

And so, just weeks before my exam, it was my luck to receive a package of immense importance. A letter and a horse shoe. The latter was a confounded nuisance in the pocket of my jacket during the exam, but since I passed, I bore it no ill-will and I treasure it yet. And the letter? That letter was my lifeline and the start of a long and regular correspondence.

Before long we had met again. I stayed with the Lanfear family near London and Viv and I went to the West End to see a film. There were long queues outside the cinema and we ended up joining the wrong queue and attending a film we had no intention of seeing, but didn't see anyway. It took us a long time to get home but, as I recall, we were at least thirty seconds inside the allotted curfew. By the time I had to take the train home we knew that we were going to see a lot more of each other.

I had taken my first bite of the apple. The Lanfears had a large Bramley tree at the end of their garden and I knew I was going to be well fed.

It was most fortunate that Viv's parents were tolerant of this student interloper. Not only had he found a new girlfriend, but he was generously welcomed into their home. Thanks to them I now had a new base from which to expand my veterinary education and during the holidays I was able to gain work experience in a modern veterinary practice near Watford.

~

Apart from being a loving and understanding girlfriend, Viv looked the part of any young man's dream of the late 1960s. She had long, blond hair and legs that embellished many a mini-skirt. With her white calf-length boots she needed but one accoutrement to be my *femme fatale*. Almost before I realised what, I had set myself a challenge that would sorely test any diffident, hormone-laden, teenaged male.

And so it was with great trepidation that I entered the anonymity of a large Liverpool department store, and headed for the bras and panties. Like most men of that era, still less callow youths, I had little nous when it came to navigating a women's lingerie department. Other men stood awkwardly on an ill-defined shoreline, nonchalantly examining their fingernails or imaginary distant vistas, whilst their female partners recklessly plunged into a mystical island of intimate female apparel. Purposefully, for I did not wish to appear furtive, I stepped across the boundary and into this realm of cardboard cut-out sirens. Pink, lacy, black, flesh, legs, busts, bosoms, bottoms, crutches, cleavages... all forbidden territory.

At such moments one comes to realise the power of one's peripheral vision. I took great pains to avoid looking directly at the photos of these scantily clad models, much as I would have liked to in different circumstances. I blurred past them, seeking out the hosiery section. I sensed the curiosity of women looking up at this clumsy little pervert invading their domain – or I imagined I did, which had the same effect on my confidence. But despite everything, I knew I wouldn't be able to live with myself if I didn't complete this mission.

Blushing and sweating profusely I fumbled through the stockings.

'Can I help you, love?' Did I detect the slightest hint of irony in the assistant's question?

'Well, I'm looking for a pair of these for my girlfriend,' I managed to stammer, holding up a pair of black fishnet stockings.

'Oh aye, and what size might she be then?' It is absolutely true for me to state here that Viv's legs are about the same length as my own. It suddenly dawned on me that I was going to have to give this assistant precisely the answer on which I imagined, in my paranoid state, she would pounce. So I did.

'She's about my size.' I can't say I looked her in the eye as I anticipated the 'that's what they all say' response. I merely got a look of pity when she put the item in a brown paper bag. Looks can deceive, but I suspect 'guilty of perversion' was written all over my blushing face.

The moment was prolonged as I fumbled for cash and then found, poor penurious student, that I had to write a cheque. Finally she had the ink-smudged document in her hand and I was at last free to scuttle off with my prize, more relieved than triumphant. It was one of the bravest things I have ever done.

Viv's response was more sympathetic, although not overwhelmingly reassuring. She wore them occasionally, just to please me, but I was never fully able to convince her of the sacrifices I had made to bring her my tribute.

The moral of this story, for every young man, is that the way to a woman's heart is not necessarily through her stockings.

CHAPTER THIRTEEN

HORSES FOR COURSES

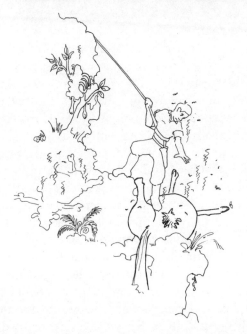

We were young, absurdly young as others liked to point out, but two years later we were married. What else is there for it when you meet your soul mate? For those two years we had not merely communicated, but communed. We were spiritually compatible and our love for each other certain. We revelled in the brief weekends we could be together and share the profundity of classical music for which we have an abiding passion. Together we had tramped the Scottish Highlands, wandered the Lakeland Fells and ridden horses along the A5.

It wasn't my choice. As part of our practical training in the first two years of university vacations we were required to work on farms, in riding establishments, dog kennels: anywhere that would broaden our experience of animal handling and husbandry. My contact with horses had been confined to a back-street riding school in Liverpool. It was a rough and tacky establishment and I learned enough about the seamy side of this colourful industry to discourage me from further equine experiences. That was until I met Viv. She had an interest in ponies, as many young girls do. Eventually her parents had acceded to her repeated requests and her persistence was rewarded with a strong-willed pony called Coffee. One of Viv's friends had a larger pony, Playboy, which shared Coffee's field.

Playboy was spoilt. He hadn't been ridden recently and was ready for action. I was to prove my manhood by following my true love on this trusty steed. Together we traversed the meadows and bridleways of Hertfordshire. But this is an overpopulated corner of an overpopulated country. Glorious tree-bound fields were all too frequently interspersed with roads bristling with traffic. It wasn't until we reached the A5, one of the largest highways feeding London, that Playboy decided he was a leader and no longer content to follow. At the same time he ascertained that while his rider may have been determined, he certainly wasn't experienced. Also the girth was loose and the saddle starting to slide. This was to be, for me, an unhappy combination of circumstances. While Viv cantered Coffee on the green verge, Playboy overtook them at full gallop with rider hanging round his neck. As that rider I was conscious that I had no control, and that I was perilously close to the lorries and cars roaring past in the opposite direction.

Fortunately when Coffee's experienced rider realised my plight, and stopped him, Playboy realised that he had won that particular race and stopped too. And anyway his lopsided cargo was starting to impede his dash for glory. I had been in mortal danger, but my sweetheart had recognised that, and the part where she showed her concern for my plight was well worth those few moments of terror.

I am one of those people who sometimes makes the same mistake twice. Although this was my last equine escapade on British soil a more scenic, but no less stimulating, repeat was to occur in New Zealand just a few years later.

~

On many backcountry stations in New Zealand, horses are still used to muster sheep and cattle in rough terrain. I regard it as a privilege to have worked during a period when there were still quite a few station hacks around, although the numbers have dropped off rapidly in recent years. Treating these animals is relatively straightforward because, like most working animals, they are un-pampered and easy to handle and their owners have a pragmatic approach to injuries and treatment. Besides, they are sheep farmers and sheep farmers are in my considered opinion the salt of the earth. I could not say that about a large percentage of the horse-owning public.

And so, one windy summer day, Viv, Brian – a friend and vet with whom I was working in a mid-Canterbury veterinary practice – and muggins drove to the remote Erehwon Station. Samuel Butler, the English author, had established this station in the mid-nineteenth century and his satire *Erehwon* ('nowhere' backwards) had been inspired by the lonely and, in those days, unexplored lands over the mountains to the west.

We hired the station horses and set off up the broad shingle bed of the mighty Rangitata River and into the shadows of the Southern Alps. The three of us slowly worked our way up the valley into the teeth of a fresh nor'wester. Brian – a man who had been brought up with horses and had a classical sense of style – erect and confident in his saddle, Viv competent and revelling in the knowledge that she had overcome my reluctance to ever mount a horse again, and me, delighting in the magnificence of the scenery and the adventure on which we were embarking. The horses were slow and plodding to my (secret) satisfaction. Viv and Brian were disappointed that they could not be cajoled into more than a brisk trot, but it was windy and the going rough. It fell on me to carry the panniers of provisions fashioned from our backpacks and they were strapped behind my saddle. I wasn't bothered about the galloping part, so was able to play the uncomplaining martyr with conviction.

Before nightfall we had reached a musterers' hut. The Watchdog hut. What powerful evocations a name brings. There it was, set in an alpine meadow, melting into background of matagouri and coprosma scrub. We hobbled the horses on the sweet grass. This is the best part – such promises ahead. We contemplated the rocky, snow-streaked peaks surrounding us and selected a spur to climb the following day. However, pennants of ragged cloud streaking from the west did not augur well. During the night the storm broke and the tin walls of our puny shelter were drummed by torrential rain. Who has not also experienced the snug refuge of a remote hut without a feeling of privilege and awe?

Although the rain had eased by dawn, our assault on the ridge was cut short by lowering cloud and we returned to the hut and prepared the horses for departure. The rain had raised the river and the weather had by now swung round to the south so we faced a cold ride back into the wind once again.

The horses, however, were now pointing homewards. It was remarkable how they were able to pick a safe route across the shingle and through the swollen strands of the braided river. There were a couple of awkward moments crossing some swift, deep water, places we could never have gone on foot. Then, as we neared the homestead, ears pricked and the pace quickened. I was about to experience the New Zealand version of my A5 incident.

A grassy flat was irresistible for the more experienced equestrians in our party and their horses needed minimal encouragement. Little did I know, but once again, unfortunately, I had picked a winner. As the others took off on a full-scale gallop I held my mount on a tight rein. Gradually I lost the battle of wills; the brisk trot became a canter. As we cantered, the panniers behind my saddle started to bounce. Dobbin was getting mixed messages. A couple of rucksacks thumping on his flanks spurred him on in no uncertain way and seemed to influence him more than my pull on the reins. In the end I had no choice but to give him his head and concentrate on retaining my seat. Just like Playboy, he was determined to win anyway. An observer would have seen two elegant riders whooping joyously across the turf, being rapidly overhauled by an indecorously clinging novice athwart an uncontrolled horse, the bulky packs flapping like wings. But Dobbin knew what he was doing. As he had sure-footedly crossed that river, so was he perfectly assured in that flight across the rough grass.

In the end it was an exhilarating episode and I can understand the fascination that these wonderful and powerful animals have held throughout history but, personally, I prefer to control my own destiny rather than entrust it to a horse.

~

Mortality spares neither weak nor powerful and the practising vet must familiarise himself with the dead as well as the quick. Perhaps the worst job that ever befell me involved a dead horse.

'Is that you, John?' Murray enquired anxiously down the phone. 'I was looking after Mrs Jabcowski's daughter's pony while she was overseas and now she's back again.'

I couldn't understand the reason for his anxiety. I didn't even know Mrs Jabcowski. If I had, maybe I would have felt the same. Murray was a kind-hearted sheep farmer, who had offered grazing on his farm for this friend-of-a-friend's nag, and now things had backfired on him.

'The pony died a week or so back. It must have run onto a waratah [metal stake] and bled to death when I found it. Now she's insisting that I get a vet's certificate,' he elucidated. It also transpired that the pony was down an offal pit.

'Could be a bit difficult to verify the cause of death after a week,' I said, 'and you'll need to get it out of the offal pit if I'm to attempt a post-mortem. Are you sure she wants to go ahead with this?' I was playing for time. I wasn't sure that I was too keen to go ahead with this, even if she was.

'You haven't met her,' replied Murray, with marked emphasis on the last pronoun. My feeble avoidance strategy was going out of the window. I faced a wrestling match with a rotten carcase on a bitterly cold winter's day.

I have never been the sort of vet whose scientific curiosity can deflect the overwhelming olfactory assault of over-ripe carcases. Some vets love to guddle around with necrotic flesh and proclaim their fascination oblivious to the retching stench of mortification. Whilst I gasp for air and try to suppress the churning of my stomach, blither spirits gather round like vultures. I had witnessed colleagues avidly grope bubbling carcases and simultaneously hold full-blown discourses concerning the pathology revealed. How could they breathe and speak in the presence of such unmitigated sensory challenge? A routine post-mortem on the freshly dead is one thing, performing the exercise on a week-old carcase another. But there was an additional deterrent to my enjoyment of the morning.

Contrary to the opinion of those who live in the winterless north of New Zealand, snow at sea level is rare even in Southland, but this happened to be one of those days. Sleet was driving against the windows even as I made arrangements with Murray. He didn't seem too keen about retrieving the carcase, but I couldn't see that that was part of my brief. I suggested he place a noose around a back leg and haul the carcase out with the winch he claimed to possess.

Slowly, allowing Murray plenty of time to complete his task, I drove to my assignation with death. There was a tractor waiting at the gate. He had tactically decided to feed me the bad news in bits. Rather than being able to drive my car to the site I was to be conveyed to the back of his farm on a tractor.

Arriving at the top of a ridge, frozen and numbed by my journey, I was greeted by the sight of the juicy back leg of a horse with gaseous bubbles adorning the ragged area whence it had separated from its body. A long rope was knotted round the fetlock. He had made an effort, but it wasn't good enough. I noticed that we were on the edge of a cliff. I tried humour.

'Couldn't you just tell her that one of its back legs fell off?'

Murray ignored me. There was one more item of bad news he had yet to convey, but in our dramatic situation I was beginning to suspect what was coming next. Most farmers dispose of dead stock down an augur-drilled pit, sealed with a removable concrete lid. Murray had an unofficial 'pit'. For many years he had tipped carcases down the limestone cliff. Growing out from this and at its base was a wilderness of concealing bush and elder scrub. Out of sight, out of mind.

'So how do you propose that I do this post-mortem?' I asked.

Minutes later I was on the end of the rope being lowered through a charnel-house littered with carcases. Body parts festooned tree branches and made ledges slippery. This was as surreal as it gets. This was one job I should have refused to do. Surely there are limits. Or are there? Farmers are used to seeing vets pull putrid calves and membranes from cows' rear ends, lance abscesses containing litres of pus, give enemas to constipated dogs. So what's the difference?

For me, personally, it's a matter of temperature. Dealing with something warm and smelly is infinitely preferable to a foetid, cold and clammy carcase. Warmth equals life: there is a purpose to your intervention and for your patient there may be a future. Death is singularly unpromising in this regard.

After about twenty metres a three-legged horse hove into sight.

It was teetering on a small ledge. Beyond, there was another drop into a veritable welter of sheep carcases. Gingerly I examined the bloated body. Indeed there was a gash where a waratah could have penetrated the jugular vein. I yelled above for a pull-up as I stepped off the gaseous carcase, and let it wheeze and slough further into the abyss.

It was all going to be an expensive exercise for Mrs J for relatively unimportant information – a test of Murray's veracity. The horse wasn't even insured. I was going to have to be very careful as to how I worded my certificate '...unable to complete a thorough autopsy... lesions consistent with death due to...'.

When I got to the top Murray asked my opinion. I wasn't going to let him off easily.

'It all looks rather suspicious to me,' I said. 'From the angle of the wound I could guarantee that someone had snuck up on that pony in the middle of the night and tried to drive a stake through its heart. Such incidents are not unheard of. There was a full moon last week. What were you doing on Sunday night?'

I was rewarded with a wry look.

Little was he to know that mine had just been a practice run.

As I reached the roadside another vet's car drew up. Mrs Jabcowski must have decided not to trust the word of Murray's vet and had recruited the services of her own, albeit he'd had to drive over a hundred kilometres for this plum job. Dr Evans was typical of a certain type of horse vet, and I was treated with the disdain characteristic of this superior form of being. He grunted in surprise at my presence, or was it a greeting?

'Fancy meeting you here, Geoff! Just follow my tracks till you get to Murray on his tractor over there,' I told him. 'You shouldn't have too much trouble once he's got you up to the ridge.'

Uncharitable pleasure can be drawn from the imagined discomfiture of certain individuals and, as far as I'm concerned, Geoff was one of them. It had been an unpromising start, but I drove away from that job with a barely suppressed feeling of glee.

CHAPTER FOURTEEN
HIGHLAND HOLIDAY

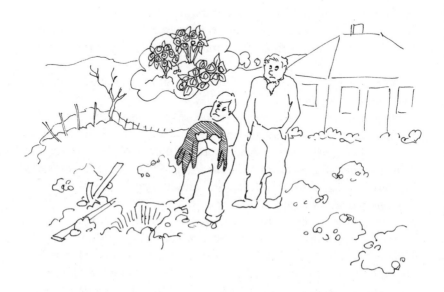

If you study a relief map of the British Isles and happen to be drawn to mountains you can't fail to notice that the most rugged part and the highest peaks are in the Highlands of Scotland. The biggest concentration of high ground is slightly east of centre, the Cairngorm mountains, a dissected plateau around 4000 feet high. This is not great by world standards and the mountains are scarcely spectacular, but there are other compensations for the visitor.

The Highlands are saturated by history of such poignancy that the ghosts of the past are closer than in most other areas of Britain, smothered as much of it is by a cloak of industry. Visiting the Highlands is a spiritual experience. Every glen has echoes of a vanished people and yet, tantalisingly, enough of a proud and distinctive culture remains to fire the imagination. The Clearances in the nineteenth century changed the face of the Highlands forever and left a void that can never be filled. The populace was dispersed, but it has stamped its culture around the world. There are now more pipe bands in New Zealand than there are in Scotland. The south of New Zealand in particular has a strong Scottish heritage focused particularly on Dunedin, a town with a distinctly Scottish feel.

A friend of ours in Southland had traced his ancestors to a ruined bothy near the Ryvoan Pass, beneath the slopes of Cairngorm. It was a startling revelation in later life to find that he had stood in the very same spot of isolated and wild beauty that Viv and I had shared, from where we gazed, as his forbears had, to Airgiod-meall, Creag a' Chalamain and other hills that they, in their ancient tongue, had named. Names, sadly, that I cannot pretend to pronounce or understand. The Gaelic diaspora will ever seek to replenish its culture from its Highland source. If I had the privilege of Highland ancestry I would be driven to explore further. We are all enriched by understanding our roots, even as we look to the future.

By the time I had reached my third summer at university I felt that I had survived the worst that academia could throw at me. Viv and I had been married for almost a year and things were going well. We both passed our exams at the end of the year and, for the first time, I had evaded the dreaded re-sits that had blighted earlier summer vacations. Seeing practice near London had been professionally rewarding, but scarcely inspiring. I wasn't training for a career in the 'concrete jungle' and Viv shared my love for wild places. It was time for us to head for the hills.

I was intrigued by letters written in *The Veterinary Record* by a vet who shared practical tips with his profession. I shall call him Mr Sinatra, but perhaps that is not his real name. Mr Sinatra ran a practice from Brigadoon, within sight of the Cairngorms. Supervising students is a chore for many veterinarians. Explaining procedures and letting them try them out can be time-consuming. On the other hand, a motivated and questioning student can clarify your justifications, provide company during what can sometimes be a lonely career, open the gates, carry your equipment and bury your dogs: of which more later. I was pleased to receive a warm response to my request to see practice and grateful that Mr Sinatra inclined to pedagogy and enjoyed showing students the ropes. With his help, Viv and I were able to rent a caravan near to his clinic.

We were based there for several weeks and while I did the rounds with Mr Sinatra, or one of his assistants, Viv worked at a local riding school.

On our free weekends we explored remote corners of the ancient granite landscape of the Cairngorms. We tramped reverentially through the Scots pines (*Pinus sylvestris*) of the Rothiemurchus Forest. Sombre green needles set off their textured trunks; yet in the dying rays of a summer evening, the delicate and surprising reds of their upper branch tips glowed. At such times, these grizzled outliers, of great age and character, emanated an almost palpable aura of mystery. What trysts, what clash of arms occurred beneath their twisted limbs? I love most trees but these disappearing remnants of a once much vaster Caledonian forest echoed the dying of an archaic way of life.

We camped out on Braeriach and woke to a brilliant dawn above a sea of silver cloud. We traversed the droving route used by the clans: the defile of the Lairig Ghru. Our imaginations were fired by the romantic ruins of the thirteenth-century castle in Loch an Eilein – though the reality of the bloody history of the Highlands should 'scotch' any notions of romance.

Meanwhile I imbibed what I could from one of the great individualists of the veterinary profession. Perhaps more even than Mike, Mr Sinatra was a conscious servant of the public. He did not spare himself in this regard, to the point of asceticism. His idea of a holiday was to spend a few days a year cutting peat. This was but one example of that legendary Scottish thrift.

Disposal of deceased dogs and cats is always a problem in veterinary practice. Despite our best efforts, not all our patients live forever. When the sad day comes, the owners have to decide what they want to do with the body of their beloved pet. Many choose to bury the pet themselves in their own garden; the problem arises when they are unable or unwilling to do this. Mr Sinatra had the smartest solution. Adjacent to his clinic there was an area of rough ground. In fact it was not only rough, but positively rocky, as I, and no doubt many generations of students, could attest. For Mr Sinatra there was no, 'What would you like to do with Fru-Fru, Mrs Sphengalis. I'm sure you've picked a lovely spot in that garden of yours?' but more, 'It would be no trouble for us to bury Jock for you, Mrs McPherson, if that is your wish.'

For the student bystander the client's choice held some significance. If the dog was a Great Dane, or a big fat Labrador, you could not help but hope that the kind offer would be declined. But, as often as not, you would soon be out there with pickaxe or crowbar. Mr Sinatra planned to turn the whole area into a rose garden and, for all I know, there could be one flourishing there now.

If Mr Sinatra could save money for himself and his clients he would. Whenever there was a lull in the work, he would be manufacturing metabolic solutions for cattle or preparing worm drenches from bulk ingredients. He was always occupied and could present an austere front to his employees should he consider them slacking. The moment his feet were heard scrunching on the gravel his two assistants, who may have been enjoying a moment of leisure after a hectic surgery, would leap up and pretend to busy themselves making calcium borogluconate solutions. They were scared of him! Here was an opinionated man of immensely strong will and physical presence. He exerted almost total control over his staff.

As a student this did not directly affect me. I was there to learn, and I picked up many useful tips and saw conditions that were unusual elsewhere; although the dynamics of that workplace were also fascinating. I realised that no matter how magic the area I could never enjoy working under such claustrophobic control. Mr Sinatra took the lyrics a step further and expected everyone 'to do it his way'.

I seemed to be getting along fine with him, but I dreaded putting a foot wrong. So far he had been very careful in his supervision as I mastered the basics of vaccinating sheep, castrating cattle, injecting dogs and so on, but, after a week or so, he gradually trusted me to do more. Then one day, as he was chatting with a client in his farmyard, he chucked his car keys to me.

'Turn the car round for me please, John.'

My feelings of glee at gaining the trust of this dour, and slightly forbidding, man were tempered by a small inner voice. I had never driven a Volkswagen before. But how could I refuse? It would have seemed feeble to request a test-drive on the open road before tackling this tiny yard. Regrettably, I suppressed my fears:

'Certainly, Mr Sinatra.'

This *was* a tiny yard, and the lock on the vehicle wasn't as tight as I had thought. After successfully traversing an arc of about ten yards I connected with the tow-bar of a wagon thoughtlessly left there by the farmer. I clutched my head in despair and shame. It would be a major understatement to say that it was embarrassing to step out of that car in front of the two witnesses, who had abruptly discontinued their conversation to watch me. Fortunately the only damage was to a headlight and my self-esteem. One could be repaired for about five pounds, and a cuddle or two from Viv would help to restore the other. But how was the forbidding Mr Sinatra going to react to my clumsiness?

As we drove away I made arrangements to pay for the damage I had caused. Five pounds was quite a lot of money for a student. And then he really surprised me:

'Never mind, John. I reckon that this is part of the price we pay for taking on students. It's fine to make mistakes sometimes, as long as we learn from them.'

Such unexpected magnanimity restores one's faith in human nature.

I thought it prudent not to relate my Norwegian escapade with the tractor to him at this stage in our relationship. Mr Sinatra firmly refused all my subsequent offers of payment. I could only present him with a well-earned bottle of whisky when I departed. It was a small token for the rich experience I had gained over a memorable summer.

CHAPTER FIFTEEN

ANTIPODEAN ANTICIPATION

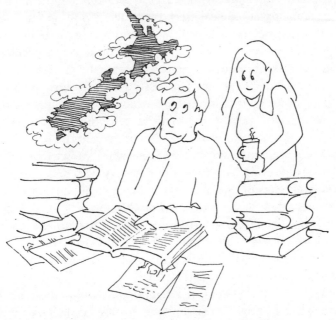

For my fifth and final year as an undergraduate I was a kept man. While Viv set off for her uninspiring daily encounter with a desk at the local building society, my mind was being filled with enormous volumes of fascinating information. The dreaded finals loomed and failure was not to be countenanced. Fortunately the course had taken a more practical direction and we were learning surgical techniques, reading radiographs, interpreting blood tests, assisting with anaesthetics, researching case histories and, in general, building on the theoretical knowledge we had painstakingly acquired in those early years. Finally, the prospects of becoming independent, making a career choice and deciding where we could live empowered us. The world would be our oyster if we could successfully negotiate the year ahead.

My only chance was to pace myself and I continued to be a

diligent, if socially unexciting student. Not for me the caffeine-soaked sprint of some of my colleagues. For them the exams were an obstacle that could be hurdled from a standing start, and two weeks of agonising effort, working in the library till the wee small hours, sufficed. The competitive element was also a factor and for some it was important to be seen indulging this passion openly. Such players would endlessly discuss esoteric topics in the hope of attaining some psychological ascendancy over a poor unfortunate who was not privy to such vital information. This sparring was an important aspect of our training. Do you defer to pointless erudition, bullshit in defence (perfectly legitimate as long as you don't suspend judgement on what passes your own lips), go away and worry about your ignorance (in which case they have won), or accept that you can't know everything, acknowledge the fact and find out more about it (the counsel of maturity)?

In a world where the sum total of veterinary knowledge is estimated to double every five years I think it is essential that veterinarians, and everyone else who derives a living from dispensing advice, give themselves permission to say 'I don't know'; as long as they then take the trouble to inform themselves. Unfortunately some sectors of the public expect their vet to know everything. More unfortunately some vets lead their clients to believe that they do, and, worst of all, some vets actually believe it.

A certain type of client enjoys attempting to exploit these weaknesses. She has the power to disrupt inter-professional relationships at her local veterinary clinic. She breeds exotic cats (or dogs). She demands instant service. She has a favourite vet; only he has the ability to gratify her whims. If he is unavailable she treats his replacement with disdain. He has immediately failed the first test by not recognising the breed of exotic mutant that Mrs Catbreeder has placed before him:

'I am surprised, Mr Largeanimalvet. Didn't you know that this is a chocolate-pointed Marquesan?' Her confidence in the said vet has been sadly compromised. Mr L tries to bring the consultation onto a clinical plane:

'Yes, but the point is he has a rather nasty abscess at the base of his tail. It looks as though he's been in a fight and picked up an infection.'

'Are you sure he hasn't been poisoned?' Ah! *Paranoia* is surfacing...

'Well there wouldn't be an abscess if he had been poisoned. Look there is pus dripping out of that hole.' This is a big mistake, Mr L. You have yet to learn that clients like Mrs C prefer a diagnosis which involves blame.

Disgruntled client, 'It looks more like a bullet hole to me. Some of the neighbours' kids have been mucking around with air rifles.'

'But if you look closely, Mrs C, you can see a couple of other skin marks. I'm sure this abscess is the result of a bite, perhaps from another cat.' (A very common occurrence.)

'I'd be far happier if Mr Felinevet was here to see Cadburyears.'

'Fair enough, he was just having a catnap [Mr L's feeble pun is sarcasm, for his own benefit, and not intoned] when I last saw him. I'll see if he's free.'

Mr L returns with Mr F, who has been briefed. He examines the cat with due obsequiousness.

'Ah, Mrs Catbreeder, these Marquies do seem to be very prone to infections.' As a clinical observation this may well be bullshit, but it is inspired bullshit because it reinforces just how special this cat is. Owners of unusual breeds revel in their pets' propensity to suffer from unusual conditions. If they don't suffer from them, they are unhappy. It's but a short step to *Munchausen by proxy*.

'We will have to be extremely careful with his anaesthetic.' (No more careful than with any other moggy, but Mrs C is lapping it up.)

'Oh, Mr Felinevet,' looking disdainfully at Mr L, 'I'd be very happy if you could deal with Cadburyears for me.'

How things proceed from here very much depends on whether the practice works as a team, or if Mr F feeds on such adulation. If he does it will be but a Pyrrhic victory and he will probably end up working by himself: a considerable disadvantage with the demands of modern veterinary practice in a world full of nutters.

~

Apart from brief forays into the Welsh hills, Viv and I mostly restricted ourselves to the confines of our small flat at the veterinary field station in Cheshire. We had a radio, a record player and textbooks for company. We were stressed, happy and focused, a heady mixture. There were a few months of effort ahead of us:

and then? There was no shortage of veterinary jobs, but closer inspection revealed that many were in depressed urban areas. The box number concealed the location. Did I really want to work in Wigan, even if the advert stipulated that they were all Christians? The denomination was of no consequence, but we did seek a rural district and I wanted to try and build as many skills on the foundation of my degree as possible. A veterinary degree is very broad. You are equipped to cope with a range of species and it seems a shame to specialise too early. After a couple of years dealing entirely with dogs and cats it takes a major effort to diverge into rural practice and vice versa. Ideally I sought a mixed practice where I could do both small- and large-animal work, and we both needed somewhere close to the wild places to feed our souls. That left out most of south England and much of the industrial Midlands. Wales and its borders, the far north of England and much of Scotland would have suited, but then an advert appeared on the university notice board.

'Viv, how would you like to go to New Zealand?'

Almost at once we were caught up in the adventure. It seemed too good to be true. New Zealand was short of veterinarians. The first New Zealand-trained vets were only just starting to emerge from Massey University, and to make up the shortfall the New Zealand government ran a scheme to entice vets from overseas. They would pay travelling expenses to New Zealand for Viv as well as me, plus a provision for furniture removal. The only condition was that we would be bonded to work for a rural veterinary club for three years.

The job vacancy was in Taranaki in a predominantly dairy practice on the slopes of Mount Egmont (now officially reverting to its more poetic Maori name of Mount Taranaki). We pored over maps. Mount Egmont was a dormant volcano over 8000 feet high and there was a 9000-foot volcano (Ruapehu) in the centre of the North Island. Between them was a wilderness of forest, forest that we would soon refer to as 'bush', a diminutive that scarcely does justice to such vast tracts. Everywhere there was high ground and, as we glanced down, the South Island looked to be a mountaineer's dream. The Southern Alps stretched its length: the white, purple and brown contours interweaving with a skirt of green plain on the east and a narrower margin to the west. For the meantime we would settle for Mount Egmont, but there were a few obstacles to surmount first.

Our preliminary interview with the New Zealand government's representative at New Zealand House in London was successful. Our assessor seemed a bit perturbed that I didn't drink much. This was just after the notorious 'six o'clock swill' had been abandoned, the era when all pubs closed at 6 pm and 'everyone' rushed down to the pub when work finished to tank up for the evening. Prodigious volumes were downed in a short space of time. New Zealand still suffers from the binge mentality this engendered. I was perturbed that he was perturbed (and also because he thought that Mount Cook was as high as the Matterhorn), but he deemed us potential immigrants even though we weren't potential alcoholics, and so I forgave him his lapse in altitudinal esoterica.

As it transpired, my trepidation of pub culture was misplaced. No one can force you to drink alcohol to excess and my moderate consumption in the local cricket team was tolerated and respected, if not emulated. It would be another decade or so before respectable women would be socially accepted in rural pubs in New Zealand, but we weren't emigrating for the pub scene.

The hardest task was to inform our parents of our decision. New Zealand is a very mobile society; young people come and go on their overseas experiences. The OE is considered a rite of passage whereas, for the majority of English people, emigration is a scarcely-contemplated option. My colleagues couldn't understand me, even the more mercenary among them who knew from the advert that my salary and working conditions would be significantly better than any they stood to gain. For our parents it was an entirely unexpected outcome from my graduation and, even though the initial term was three years, they expected the worst: that this would be a permanent move.

Emigration is, for a reflective person, one of the ultimate tests of character. We did not have the maturity to handle the wrench from our families in the most tactful manner, and there was initially considerable bitterness on their part about the inexplicable decision we had made. Time is a great healer. My parents-in-law have been frequent visitors to this beautiful country, and I was touched when after twenty-five years my father informed me that I had made the right move, something we weren't sure of ourselves till we had been many years in our adopted country. Emigration can tear you apart, it is dangerous medicine: not to be taken lightly.

CHAPTER SIXTEEN

AN IRISHMAN, A YORKSHIREMAN AND A DUTCHMAN

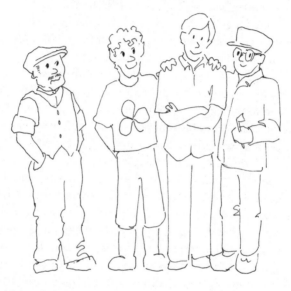

It would be dishonest to claim that I breezed through my finals, but my performance was adequate; hence seeing my name on the notice board in the right place was a cause for sweet relief rather than wild exultation. There was a lot to be done in a few days. We hadn't been tempted to finalise any travel arrangements because, without the certainty that I had passed, we felt we would have been tempting fate. Less than two weeks after graduating we were on a plane to Auckland and two weeks later, in late July 1973, I was calving cows in Taranaki.

It wasn't till we arrived in Auckland that the enormity of what we had done began to sink in. This was an alien landscape. So frequently we had been told that New Zealand is very English. True, a *similar* language is shared, but these are two very different societies. Moreover, those observers would have to have been architecturally, botanically and topographically dyslexic.

First impressions can take a long while to shake off. Some people arrive here and love the country at first sight. They know they have come to the land of their dreams. For us there was a suppressed feeling of disappointment. Suppressed because neither of us dared voice it, because we feared our judgement was impaired by our jetlagged state, because we had no option than to accept our fate. For a while three years seemed like a long time.

Just look at those houses with their tin (corrugated iron) roofs. In Britain corrugated iron is only used on farm sheds and shacks, it doesn't last at all in the corrosive atmosphere of the big cities, but here it is entirely practical, versatile and colourful. The whole place has an air of impermanence, because it has only been settled since the 1830s. There is a history: a fascinating history of pioneering settlement, but forget the Roman remains, and the twelfth-century cathedrals. Try to ignore the ghastly wild-west signage festooning the approach to each rural town. This country is only just starting to realise its own past and teach its own history in its schools. A generation of brilliant New Zealand historians are only now beginning to explore and interpret this past for us. The bush has been ripped out to make way for farm land and there is little biodiversity. Few wild flowers in the roadside verges – willows, pines and macrocarpas (Monterey Cypress) with boxthorn hedges, that seems to have been the limit of the settlers' plantings: robust, functional, uninspiring. But wait till you see the bush: so much of it destroyed, but so much now preserved in National Parks and reserves. In time you will see a quantum leap in imaginative landscape design and amenity plantings. Slowly you have to learn that you are not going to like everything, why did you want to come in the first place? Look at the unpopulated countryside; see the friendly, smiling people. The potential here is enormous. And so it has proved. The New Zealand of today is very different to that we saw out of Peter's car window as he drove us south to Taranaki.

Peter was a Yorkshireman who had emigrated eight years earlier. It is interesting to observe the social baggage that English immigrants bring with them to their adopted country. Peter proudly acclaimed his working-class origins. This may seem pointless in a country which conspicuously lacks class boundaries, but he had had a 'guts full' of dealing with the 'nobs' in a Norfolk practice, one of the main reasons he and his wife had decided to leave. The problem was that he immediately identified me as an ex-public schoolboy, the way English people do. For him that spelt privilege, snobbery, the old-school-tie system. My parents had paid for my education, whereas he had made his way through the school of hard knocks. Because, at the age of eleven, I hadn't been able to pick that of the three: a tractor, a table and a cow, the tractor is the odd one out because it hasn't got legs, I had failed my eleven-plus and any chance of entering grammar school. I was lucky that my parents had refused to consign me to the educational scrapheap that the local comprehensive school would have been for me. But I was tired of fighting this resentment of the English public school system. I wasn't particularly enamoured of it myself, but to come to New Zealand and be branded a willing accomplice was a bit rich. I was going to have to gain Peter's respect the hard way.

Despite this undercurrent, relationships were very cordial and the other two vets were openly welcoming. Sean was charming in the way only Irish people can be, and my boss was a warm-hearted and kindly Dutchman, Alex. It was going to be a good team for an apprehensive new graduate about to start his career.

For a few days I was taken round the practice, introduced to farmers, and given a brief insight into their farming systems. It was the end of July (equivalent to the end of a northern hemisphere January) and yet it wasn't that cold. For those who take the term 'antipodes' literally it comes as some surprise to realise that New Zealand occupies latitudes comparable to those of Italy. With its softly temperate climate it is a farmer's dream. Nowhere else in the world is superior for pasture production. If you can grow grass well, milk, beef, lamb and wool will follow. Even during the coldest months animals can be wintered outside without the expense of housing. New Zealand farmers are able to compete globally, despite their long distance from markets, because of their efficient management of this low cost, grass-based industry.

Most of the dairy farms produce milk destined for export in the form of cheese, milk powder and other by-products such as casein and rennet. Only a small volume is for local consumption. Consequently there are very few herds that milk round the year, most are seasonal suppliers. The cows' natural cycle of birth in spring, milk through summer, dry-off in autumn and rest in winter is the most efficient to adopt. It follows the growth pattern of grass. Peak grass growth in spring coincides with maximum milk production for the growing calf. This was why I was needed so soon.

In Taranaki, July is the month when the cows start calving. Over the next two months nearly every cow in our district would calve. A large number, even if a small percentage, would need veterinary assistance. Springtime in dairy practice in New Zealand is hectic. I was commencing at the deep end. My apprehension wasn't going to last long.

By the end of the calving season Sean reckoned that we had each assisted at least a hundred cows to give birth. These dystocias had been hard going at first. I knew that I could call on a colleague for assistance and to start with I did. On one occasion I was unable to straighten the neck on a calf with its head back. The cow was lying down, squashing any free space and I felt that I had reached my limit. Peter answered my call for assistance over the radio-telephone and got stuck in straightaway. He was having a hard task judging by the accompanying sweat, grunting and odd expletive as he rolled around seeking purchase on the head of the calf. I was secretly gratified that my difficulties seemed to have been justified. Finally he had the head up and soon a new-born calf sucked the cool night air.

'How did you do that?' I asked innocently.

'I kept on f***ing trying,' was the stern reply. (He didn't need to add 'you soft little public schoolboy, twat'; it was implicit in his tone). From then on I managed every calving without further assistance. As a vet the buck has to end with you. You have to provide the solution; there is no referring to specialists and, really, my colleagues were by now busy enough themselves without having to do my job.

One of the problems with big herds is that farmers, too, are under stress over spring. With herds of only twenty or thirty cows, as in Mike's practice back in the Yorkshire Dales, it was different. If Daisy was due to calve Jonty Capstick would sit up all night waiting for trouble. The situation I am about to describe scarcely happens in Britain.

The average herd size in Taranaki was a hundred. The farmer needed his sleep. He couldn't stay sleepless for two months, so there was the odd cow that missed the system. Let's say old 73 starts to calve one Saturday afternoon. When George Brown does his nightly check she is away from the main mob in a gully. He misses seeing her. All night she strains to no avail, the calf is a breech (coming backwards but with the back legs tucked forwards) and the calf is wedged in her pelvic canal. In this case not even the calf's tail is showing. Around dawn she gives up trying. It is pouring with rain.

George misses her again on his morning rounds; he has a later calving date for her anyway, so he doesn't notice her. There is nothing to see at a cursory glance and there are three other cows requiring his immediate attention. Cows are tough, stoical, and naturally resistant to uterine infections. It's not till Monday night that he sees number 73 with her tail out, straining. By now the calf has been dead and cooking away at body temperature inside her for forty-eight hours. It is blown up with the gases of putrefaction and her placental fluids have dried. 73 has become what is known as a 'fizzer', so much more expressive than the prosaic 'emphysematous calf' of my exam papers. This is no academic exercise. She's really straining now. Time to call the vet.

'Vet base to Vet 4.'

'Vet 4 receiving.'

'George Brown has got a cow he'd like you to look at.'

'OK, what seems to be the problem?'

It helps to be able to mentally prepare for the next little escapade and run through the list of possibilities.

'She's straining and she hasn't calved. She smells a bit, too. He'll try and get her to the shed, but she's a bit reluctant to move.'

Blast! Only one possibility. Wish I'd never asked. Now I've got twenty minutes driving time to contemplate one of the most awful jobs a vet has to do.

'Thanks a lot, if you haven't heard from me in a couple of hours send out the ambulance with oxygen and a gallon of rosewater.'

Fortunately George has got her to the shed. At least we'll have light, a clean working area, and lashings of hot water.

'Hello, George, my name's John. I'm the new vet.'

'Gidday, John. Welcome aboard. How long have you been out from home?' They often referred to Britain as 'home', these older generation New Zealanders. They had been brought up on British history, British literature and were generally well imbued with

British culture. They (mostly) understood British humour, while their children laughed at the American stuff. A higher proportion of New Zealanders had been killed in two world wars fighting on Britain's side than those of any other colony. During the Great War over seven per cent of all New Zealand men between the ages of eighteen and forty-five died in the service of His Majesty. The ties with Britain were very strong, but Britain's destiny with the European Union has changed that, and Britain is no longer 'home'.

George is an older man. Mid fifties. Been through the desert campaigns of the Second World War. He has an open smiling face.

After a preliminary procrastinatory chat we were down to business. 73 was crouching and straining as I put my well-lubricated arm into her dry, dry vagina. I flicked the calf's tail out.

'You're making progress, lad.'

But that was about all the progress I was going to make. There really is no easy solution in some of these cases. A caesarean is usually out of the question. Most cows with rotten calves in them die of peritonitis within a day or two of the operation. Occasionally a foetotomy can be performed and the calf sectioned with special cutting wire or finger blades and removed in pieces. In selected cases the cow is put on a stiff course of antibiotics and revisited a few days later. Autolysis will by then have progressed further and a broth of stinking bones, skin, teeth and miscellaneous unrecognisable organs can be raked out. Cows are tough and many will survive. However, for cow 73 there was no choice.

'I'm afraid her uterus has ruptured, George. She hasn't got a hope. All this rotten gloop is going into her abdominal cavity. She's going to die of toxic shock and peritonitis. It would be kinder to shoot her now.' I felt a failure, even though it was no fault of mine.

George understood the situation at once.

'You've tried your best lad. She'll be right.' There: another expression never heard these days, but harking right back to the pioneering past. You had to make do. As long as you'd done your best what was the point of stressing out, looking to blame and even seeking legal redress – the modern solution? I found George's attitude comforting. It didn't help old 73; the outcome was unsatisfactory for everyone, but we had done what we could. Later there was widespread castigation of the 'she'll be right' mentality, perhaps more in the context of poor standards of workmanship, but to me, at this stage in my career, they were words of comfort.

I was warming to the New Zealand farmers. In the main they were pragmatic, honest, resourceful and, above all, friendly. As many were only first, second or third generation immigrants they had some understanding of the difficulties of leaving 'home' and they were generally appreciative that vets would want to come out and work with them.

Taranaki had experienced a severe drought in 1973 and that spring was very hard on stock, with feed deficits on many farms. I was to hear 'she'll be right' and 'where there's live ones there's dead ones' rather a lot in my first few months as a vet.

CHAPTER SEVENTEEN

WHAT DO YOU THINK ABOUT NEW ZEALAND?

> Into my heart an air that kills
> From yon far country blows:
> What are those blue remembered hills,
> What spires, what farms are those?
>
> That is the land of lost content,
> I see it shining plain,
> The happy highways where I went,
> And cannot come again.
>
> A.E. Housman, **A Shropshire Lad**

Almost the first request of any visitor to New Zealand was for an opinion of the place. Before a celebrity even had a chance to collect his/her bags from the airport terminal, a TVNZ microphone would be thrust at them with the standard:

'So what do you think about New Zealand?'

They could be tetchy, 'Look, I've had a twenty-four hour flight and, to be honest, I can't tell just at the moment'.

Sarcastic, 'Our landing was delayed by fog, but you have some of the finest tarmac in the world'.

Or fawning, 'This is a wonderful little country, you have such pretty scenery and smiling, friendly people – no wonder you folks here call it Godzone'.

Even if the latter was the response elicited, it didn't seem to register. The same question would be paraded out to each new visitor.

Can you imagine the average Parisian asking what you think of Paris? He doesn't give a *merde* what you think. As long as it suits him, your opinion is immaterial. This enquiry is seldom heard these days, thank goodness. New Zealanders have more self-belief and confidence in their own identity. Some of this change in attitude was brought about by the shock of having these national insecurities dissected and exposed by British author Austin Mitchell in *The Half-gallon, Quarter-acre, Pavlova Paradise*, a book which was published around the time of our arrival. It created quite a stir. No one enjoys having their weaknesses lampooned, and there was a fair amount of anti-British resentment as a result.

But the Kiwi of thirty years ago needed that little bit of reassurance. Though we weren't exactly celebrity status, our opinions were still sought. It wasn't an easy question to answer. It was almost like a health enquiry.

'Gidday, John, and how're you doing?' No one really wants to know unless it's 'wonderful', 'box of birds' or some similar enormously positive reply. What did we think of New Zealand? True, the people were smiling and friendly, the scenery was not exactly pretty – a word I would reserve for roses round the porch of a thatched cottage – but often majestic and spectacular. But there was no easy answer for us because we were wrestling with an affliction that has plagued immigrants down the ages: homesickness. How can you be homesick in paradise?

Homesickness is like cancer. No one wants to know you've got it. Even the most sympathetic person can't help. It's something you have to fight yourself, or endure till the worst symptoms have passed. Unlike cancer, time tends to heal, although there will always be some scars. Immigration is a trade-off. You are not going to find that your new country has the best of everything. You may have superb countryside, but your freedom to roam it is restricted by a lack of footpaths. There may be easy parking, but the streets are wide and lack the quaintness and character of a town that has evolved before the requirements of motor vehicles. You may have left your mother-in-law 12,000 miles away, but you miss your Mum's cooking; your wife may be glad to have escaped *your* Mum's cooking, but she can't forgive you for dragging her away from *her* Mum. Immigration is a true test of character.

Since my dear mother-in-law may well read this, I have to emphasise that these are examples only. The immigrant may have gained a new country, but there is the fear that an old one has been lost. One that on reflection may not have been as undesirable as imagined.

> 'Winds of the World, give answer! They are whimpering to
> and fro–
> And what should they know of England who only England
> know?

Rudyard Kipling knew his stuff. Immigration is an opportunity to grow: not merely to branch into a new country, but explore the roots of your own culture and let them grow deeper. The cultural bonds between New Zealand and Britain are strong because generations of British immigrants have nurtured them. New Zealanders avidly consume English literature, absorb BBC-sourced television, understand and share British humour. In an area of minority taste, dear to both Viv and me, British music receives an airing on the New Zealand Concert programme at least equal to the equivalent station in Britain. Why would New Zealanders be interested in the exquisite music of Elgar, Vaughan Williams, Holst, Bax and others? Why is there a statue of Robbie Burns in the centre of Dunedin and the haggis still ritually addressed in traditional style? Why are book club mailings seemingly obsessed with Celtic and Anglo-Saxon history? We all have a deep fascination with our origins, but immigration adds poignancy to the search. Hordes of New Zealanders, Australians and Americans scour the graveyards of Britain each year, probing for their origins.

In one defining moment I recall driving around a road in the back-blocks of Taranaki. In a distance of hazy spring air the bright snow cone of its mountain floated above the intervening ridges. On the radio a piece of music I had never previously heard: the superb mezzo of Janet Baker and her meltingly lovely rendition of Elgar's *Sea Pictures*. To the musical purist this may be a flawed work but, for me, since that moment, it has been arrestingly moving. I sat in my car trying to comprehend this extreme juxtaposition. The tree ferns and snow-clad volcano were a beautiful visual contrast to the waves of very English music that washed through my mind. The scene became alien. The music called me to acknowledge my own heritage.

In reality, good music has universal appeal. The emotions that well are as much about time as place. For me Elgar evokes a fantasy of Edwardian England that no longer exists: something that perished on the Somme and in the mud of Passchendaele. For me such music may trigger a poignant fantasy trip whereas another may be prompted to recall a jaunty summer picnic by the bandstand: a memorable bratwurst washed down by a cheeky Pinot Noir. I am saddened that, for the vast majority of people, music of such all-consuming elegance, beauty and passion means absolutely nothing at all.

First generation immigrants have to accept that they may always feel torn, but as with any of life's trials they will be the richer for meeting the challenge and overcoming it or deflecting it to their advantage. As you will see, we, like many immigrants, had to physically return to our roots before we knew that our initial instinct to move had been right for us.

So, what do I think of New Zealand? It's difficult to say, but on the whole emigrating was painful and immigrating has been immeasurably enriching. With time the pangs of homesickness disappear. We have learned to revere our roots and embrace the excitement of discovering the new. New Zealand has been a wonderful place in which to raise our children. Sorry if there are too many words. I could say a whole lot more, but we'd better get back to the job in hand.

~

Faint echoing voice: 'Ah, the Great War! It really touched you, my son. Don't hold it back.'

'I will never get those images out of my mind, it smashed our heritage. You and your fellow artists did your job almost too well. The collective consciences of the millions who were never there will be forever fired by your inspiration.'

'Not if you don't work at it. Your English master imbued you with your love of Siegfried Sassoon, Wilfred Owen and Rupert Brooke. He planted the seed. Great television programming made you aware of our holocaust; sepia images stutter in your mind; strains of Holst swell your heart and sent you on your own journeys of musical discovery. The Great War was a furnace where new talent was forged. For some of us the trauma and disillusionment were so profound that our creative skills were prematurely stilled: the final elegiac utterances among our finest works. Without that overwhelming tragedy we may, as preceding generations of artists, have bared our souls, but the message might not have reached you. The pathos of war magnified our talent.'

'How can you say that? Alfred Housman was writing about an idyllic and unattainable past even before the Great War. Nostalgia has ever been part of our culture.'

'But for you *The Shropshire Lad* only came alive through George Butterworth. You discovered the rare musical jewels he bequeathed us all before he was cut down in his prime on the Somme. That war added a sublime piquancy to our art. Similarly, your young New Zealanders are inspired by the catastrophe of Gallipoli. It matters not whence this feeling comes, but it is important that you feel and retain those links with the past. It is important that generations to come have the capacity to be moved by literature and music: for they are the outlets for great sorrow and joy. We must remove from this present spiritual desert of commercialism, for there is no beauty here. Nobleness, elegance, love, beauty. Revere them. Without them life is dull and brutish. Bring up your children to enjoy the fruits of civilisation that they themselves might perpetuate it. Plant the seed, plant the seed, plant the seed...'

CHAPTER EIGHTEEN

WHAT'S IN A WORD?

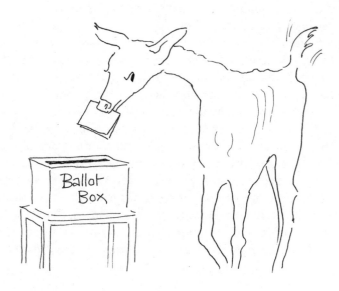

Apart from calving cows, a large portion of that first spring in Taranaki was spent treating cows for 'milk fever'. Milk fever mostly affects cows as they come into milk after calving, so the first part of the name is apt. The fever refers to the brief period of incoordination, compulsive chewing and frothing at the mouth that may accompany the onset of the illness. However, in most cases, the affected cow is not observed till she is down and unable to get up, or has even become unconscious. 'Fever' is therefore a misnomer. In fact, most cows rapidly become hypothermic once they have gone down. The reason for this complex of symptoms is a lack of circulating blood calcium.

As everyone knows, milk is rich in calcium. Suddenly, as the cow comes into milk, her system has to cope with a massive output of calcium. She can only do this by mobilising calcium reserves from her bones. As modern cows have been bred for maximum milk production the fine balance can be easily disturbed, particularly in older and more productive cows. The blood calcium deficiency results in generalised muscular weakness. Even the involuntary muscles in the intestines, bladder and uterus are affected.

Reversing these symptoms with a bottle of calcium in the vein is one of the 'miracles' of veterinary science. I recall seeing a cow unconscious with milk fever, flat out on her side, with a prolapsed uterus extending a couple of feet behind her. A uterine prolapse not uncommonly accompanies milk fever, because the uterus loses tone, becomes flaccid, and flops out. Replacing a prolapsed uterus can be a supreme physical challenge requiring veterinary savvy, and a strong back and arms. Success is helped, in good measure, by that legendary bovine resilience to injury and infection. With luck, both participants will emerge from the contest alive.

This cow had calved one clear, frosty night and was not found by the farmer till daylight. Her uterus, still wrapped with placental membranes, was frozen to the ground. I removed the protective placenta and replaced the prolapse while the farmer ran the calcium solution I had set up into her jugular vein. Within the space of a few minutes she sat up, belched, defecated (her bowels starting to move under the influence of the calcium), urinated and stood up. She was a bit wobbly on her feet to start with, but an hour later she was eating and, apart from a mud stain along her side, indistinguishable from the rest of her mob.

Before the discovery that calcium deficiency was the cause of milk fever empirical treatments were used. One is reminded of the James Herriot 'worm in t' tail'. By cutting the end off the tail, it was believed that the causative worm had been removed and the cow would recover. Mild cases do sometimes recover spontaneously, because the milk (calcium) output from a sick cow ceases. But in the case of tail amputation cause and effect are being confused, although a raw tail stump banging against a concrete floor may have been a powerful inducement to stand if at all possible! Another, more successful, treatment was to inflate the teats with air using a special pump and seal the teat ends with tape. This often worked, albeit slowly, because it stopped the flow of milk, but it was not nearly as dramatic as the response seen from rapidly restoring those levels with intravenous calcium borogluconate.

For every success there is a downside. For vets the problem with the milk fever and calcium story is the expectation that a miracle can be wrought for every downer cow. There are other reasons for cows to 'go down'. Cows which have liver damage from facial eczema (a liver disease caused by fungal toxins) or are just too thin from a difficult winter, will not respond to calcium no matter how much is put in. This is a problem for the new vet. It takes a while to gain farmers' trust.

'But Alec was here only yesterday to one exactly the same and it got up straight after he gave it a bottle of calcium.'

'Yes, but I don't think that this one is milk fever, Mark. You've already given her three bottles under the skin and she hasn't responded. If you look at her membranes here you can see she's a bit yellow. In fact she's got a yellow tinge even on the skin of her udder. That's jaundice and the most likely reason is liver damage, probably from facial eczema. I think the kindest thing would be to put her out of her misery. She's too weak to pull through now.'

Sometimes I felt more like a public executioner that spring, but I was gaining a lot of basic experience. I never squatted beside a downer cow, but rolled her onto her side and sat on her as I trickled the calcium in. It paid to keep your bum warm on a chill, and often wet, Taranaki dawn.

Milk fever, grass staggers, bloat, circling disease, woody tongue, red water, scours, ill-thrift are all descriptive terms for the conditions commonly encountered on farms. Names that have the ring of stockmanship about them; words associated with the similarly quaint-sounding occupation of animal husbandry. As veterinary medicine advanced, appellations became more scientific and lost their romance. Facial eczema, leptospirosis, campylobacteriosis belong to this next tier, but there is farmer resistance. 'Hypocalcaemia' will never replace 'milk fever' and 'prolapsed uterus' will always struggle against 'bearings'. Campylobacteriosis (a major cause of abortion in sheep) just a few years after being upgraded from vibriosis has become 'campy'.

Salmonella Brandenburg has in a couple of seasons become a major scourge of livestock in the lower South Island. The name Brandenburg conveys an image of flowing music, but the reality is more of flowing bowels and unwelcome borborygmi (and abortion in pregnant stock). This is one disease whose bite is worse than its

Bach. Within a few months of its isolation from aborting ewes we were fielding calls for information about 'this 'ere Thunderbird'. It was rather a shame that this local variant never caught on, 'Thunderbird' being far more portentous than Brandenburg; but that is the price we pay for improving educational standards.

The rich veterinary lexicon is ripe for the evolution of similar malapropisms. New Zealand was the first country in the world to embrace women's suffrage, but a few years ago I was given to understand that it had extended further.

'John, it's Dave here. I wonder if you could come and have a look at an emancipated hind for me?'

No, it wouldn't do to make a joke of it. Dave was one of the most progressive deer farmers in the district. But it would pay to establish precisely what we were talking about.

'How long has she been like this, Dave?'

'A few days, she's losing condition rapidly.'

Sure enough, when I turned up on the farm, there was the *emaciated* hind.

One of the biggest seasonal tasks facing veterinarians in sheep practice is to check that the rams going to serve the forty million ewes each autumn are capable of doing their job. Most of this is by a process of carefully feeling the scrotum and its contents for lumps that could indicate infection or injury, undersized testicles, scrotal hernias and indeed any other defects that could render them infertile: a process universally known as palpation to all but the intransigent few who want their rams 'palpitated'. It thrills my heart to reveal this.

As farming knowledge deepens and progresses, I never cease to be impressed by the readiness with which modern farmers take up new knowledge and technology. A few years back worm drenches were administered to lambs as a three-weekly routine. Monitoring of the level of worm infestation is now widely used and drenches spared for strategic occasions. Along with increasing farmer awareness has come a familiarity with the different internal parasites responsible for loss of condition or deaths in their stock. This is one circumstance where the Latin is easier than the anglicised versions. It is easier to refer to an 'Ostertagia' problem than one caused by the 'thin-necked stomach worm' and perhaps 'Haemonchus' rather than 'Barber's Pole worm'. After all they are mostly microscopic and can hardly be seen by the naked eye. How concerning then for the farmer who had a humungous worm problem.

'John, there's Eddie Calvert on the line and he reckons he's got a humungous problem, I'll put him through.'

'Hello, Eddie, what's up?'

'I reckon I've got that humungous problem.'

The lack of an indefinite article preceding the adjective alerted me that humungous was, at least in Eddie's mind, a specific condition.

'I drenched my lambs three weeks ago and some of them are still scouring.'

The penny dropped. Eddie suspected he had a problem with Haemonchus. It is indeed a worm that can cause humungous trouble.

And so to the last tier, the names that frighten off all but the most intrepid. Quite commonly we see sheep and occasionally calves that suffer from a thiamine (vitamin B1) deficiency. The rumen is a large stomach, common to all ruminants, a vast vat of bacteria and protozoa on which they rely to break down their diet. A change in the chemistry of the rumen can occur with sudden dietary change, such as when sheep are moved off dry hill country onto lush pasture. This alters the rumen microflora, one consequence being impaired thiamine production. Thiamine is essential for efficient nervous function and a deficiency manifests as damage to the brain cortex. Affected sheep press their heads against fences, become blind and deaf and may go into convulsions. Remarkably, this can be reversed if thiamine is given by injection in the early stages. The characteristic lesions caused to the brain designate the disease Cerebrocortical necrosis: CCN for those who love acronyms. When I diagnosed this in old Bill's sheep he wasn't too impressed with the name, although he did like the fact that most of his hoggets recovered. In his long life he had never heard of it, though no doubt he had seen sheep with similar symptoms. What else could he have called it? An alternative scientific name is Polioencephalomalacia (PE), not to be confused with Focal Symmetrical Encephalomalacia (FSE), a totally different disease of sheep which can cause similar symptoms. Both are relatively common conditions, but their names impede familiarity. If only they had been recognised by farmers a century ago and given a catchy epithet like 'brainrot' we'd all have thought we knew what we were talking about. But then how would we have differentiated between PE brainrot and FSE brainrot?

Maybe there will be a small bastion of knowledge that we vets can retain as our own special preserve, but the words will have to become bigger yet. The new generation of farmers is catching onto the jargon fast.

CHAPTER NINETEEN

I DON'T LIKE CRICKET: I LOVE IT. YEAH!

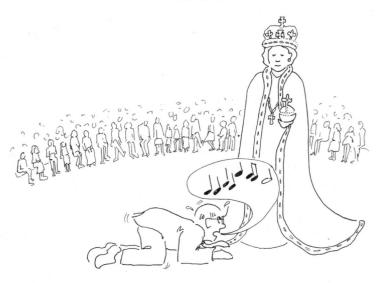

As spring turned to summer, the pressure of work eased. Mount Taranaki renounced his cloak of mist more frequently and presided over a brighter and more benign landscape. We, who laboured in his shadow, reverted to a one-in-four after-hours duty roster. There was more time for recreation.

I know that Holland does field a cricket team of sorts, but Alec was typical of most of his race. He had no interest whatsoever in cricket whereas Sean, Peter and I would often spend time in the nets after work. Sean was a precise batsman, with a mathematical bent. His love of the game drew on the accompanying statistical analysis. Indeed his other love was soccer and he would weekly note down British football results off the radio – all that 'Tranmere Rovers, nil... Birmingham Bonkers, seven' stuff. He had total recall of screeds of useless information that I would have found worrying to acquire in case it cluttered up the recesses of my tiny mind; but his was a mind born to research and Sean, after many happy years in Taranaki, eventually moved into more academic realms.

Peter was an elegant and dashing batsman. Before I could draw any incorrect assumptions from this talent he was quick to assert that in Yorkshire cricket is definitely a working class game, and that without doubt he sided with the 'players' and not the 'gentlemen'.

As for me, I had always had a passion for the game. I had spent many summer afternoons on the school playing-fields lapping up the commentary on one of those new-fangled transistor radios as our team awaited their turn to bat. John Arlott, peerless commentator, painted such evocative word-pictures in his West Country drawl. Who could not fail to love the game when introduced to it by such a master? What matter that Bill Lawry was grinding on to yet another relentlessly boring century if you found out who had planted the chestnut trees at the Vauxhall Road end of the ground, why, and when? Here was a game superficially simple, yet of enormous depth and complexity. A game rich in culture, history and imagery. Five days of test cricket were five days of oscillating drama that changed the colour of our lives. At the end of each lesson we would eagerly catch up with the progress of our team, our imaginations enriched by powerful word associations. Dark green, light green, extra cover, white flannel, red stain, willow crack, gentle applause, rain… dream on. My passion was great. Perhaps it did not matter that my talent did not match it.

Later in summer the workload in the practice, which was involved with dairy cows at least ninety per cent of the time, dropped still further as the cows, released from the trials of spring, sleeked out on juicy pastures. Alec nobly babysat while the three cricketers in his crew went to see an important game at the delightful ground at Pukekura Park in New Plymouth. Here, in a natural amphitheatre surrounded by bush and serenaded by cicadas, we had several enjoyable outings. Peter seemed to be forgetting my public school origins.

I don't know what Alec thought about our cricketing interests, for he was a true gentleman who would never speak ill of anyone. Like so many trusting people he was also extremely gullible, so easy to gull, indeed, that we only stooped to it when the occasion was irresistible.

Alec was also, for someone so competent and regularly dealing with the public, extremely shy. After many years in New Zealand, and being married to a New Zealander, he was due to become one himself. For British immigrants this was a fairly simple formality. After two years' residency you could post off your five dollars and, short of a criminal record, the honour was yours. But it was not so easy for those from 'alien cultures', as we made Alec well aware. People from outside the British Commonwealth had to swear fealty to Her Majesty at a special ceremony. Alec was not too keen on this. For a start, he wasn't convinced that every British citizen would be prepared to do the same and he contended, quite rightly, that the accident of being born under the Union Jack was no guarantee of loyalty. He had a point but, as we pointed out, rules are rules.

At this stage in history the British Royal family hadn't done too much wrong to blot their copybook, or if they had it wasn't yet public knowledge. Indeed a Royal face on a women's magazine was a guaranteed selling point to an adoring New Zealand public. Alec was politely cautious about offending the strong and recently-acquired sensitivity to all criticism of royalty that his younger vets now overtly displayed. In his presence we would explore hitherto unlikely topics such as Her Majesty's latest frock, and applaud Prince Philip's indiscretions about slitty-eyed people. In the latter case we would, of course, extend a mock sympathy to other foreigners, perhaps even those of Dutch extraction, who might be offended.

I think it was Sean who discovered that Alec was tone deaf.

'I wouldn't worry too much about the oath part, Alec,' he said.

'What do you mean?' asked Alec, hesitating. He had detected a troubling note in Sean's suggestion.

Sean enlightened him: 'Well all you have to do when taking the oath is lie back and think of Holland. I reckon having to sing 'God Defend New Zealand' in front of witnesses will be infinitely worse.'

'You're joking,' Alec stammered.

'I wish I was,' said Sean, upping the ante, 'but several people have failed and had to re-apply for their citizenship just recently. It can be quite inconvenient, not to say expensive; like those people who take forever to get their driving licence.'

Peter joined in, 'Ah, but did you see that recent article in *Truth*?' quoting a rag that no one of average intelligence would take seriously, but which was eminently suitable for lining the bottom of cat cages.

'What about it?' enquired Alec, by now visibly alarmed.

'Apparently they're only charging half price if you have to re-apply.' This was a devious attempt to buttress the veracity of the whole preposterous edifice we had fabricated by defusing the situation ever so slightly.

We would play this out for quite a while to see how many cards we could add to the house of fiction before it tumbled. Alec always took it in good grace. He even played along a bit when the light dawned. He had a great sense of humour.

Alec duly obtained his citizenship without having to expose his tonsils and without recourse to the ruse that we had suggested – slipping a fifty-dollar note into his driving licence ('as means of ID, you understand') before the ceremony. The irony of this may be lost on someone who does not appreciate that New Zealand is one of the least corrupt countries in the world. Although I have been upbraided for occasional bouts of cynicism, I suspect that this is a fair assessment.

~

I have always been impressed with the opportunities for continuing education that are available for vets in New Zealand. Soon after we arrived I was sent off to a conference, held in a pleasant setting near Rotorua. The profession is very small in New Zealand. Even today there are just 650 practising vets, so there is considerable collegial cordiality. I was used to a more hierarchical British system, and therefore amazed when on the afternoon of registration, as the delegates were assembling, an older man approached me and asked if I wanted to make up a tennis foursome with a couple of his friends. He introduced himself and we commenced to play. Unremarkable you might think, but I subsequently found him to be the current president of the New Zealand Veterinary Association. I tried to imagine the equivalent incumbent of the Royal College of Veterinary Surgeons, Nigel Pilkington Gobstrode-Browne, or whatever his name was, being able or willing to cross social barriers so easily and welcome a young upstart in such a friendly manner. That is the New Zealand way. The easy informality was totally at variance with the traditions of my own upbringing, but I warmed to it immediately.

I felt the same when the New Zealand Prime Minister of the day, Bill Rowling, sat in an aeroplane seat behind me on a routine internal flight: no fuss or flannel. It wasn't just my profession: the whole of New Zealand was a small, friendly and privileged club, and we wanted to join it. We paid our five dollars and became New Zealand citizens. As loyal British subjects of Her Majesty I recall that it was cheaper for us than for Alec.

CHAPTER TWENTY

ALPINE ADVENTURE

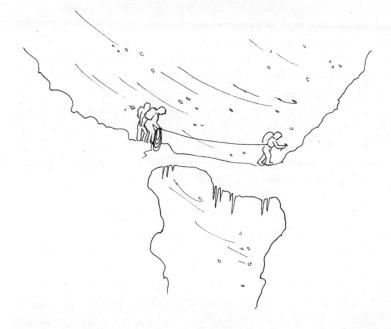

It was inevitable that we would be drawn to the looming presence of Mount Taranaki. On many weekends we had driven up the road, tunnelled through his dense skirt of enormous trees, to its end at Dawson Falls. Here a stream cascaded over a wedge of frozen magma, one of the lava flows that raked down through the forest from the cone above. From there, it seemed, we were drawn ever upwards by an exotic array of botanically-layered successions. We inhaled the cool, damp air of the alpine forest, pushed past a shrubland of hebe and leatherwood. Pressing on, through tussock grass and showy alpine plants, we would gratefully accept a bed of patchy herbfield and sprawl out, resting our limbs, and preparing ourselves for the last 1700 feet of slog over loose volcanic scoria. Viewed from the summit of this almost perfect cone the circular hem of dark forest skirt strikingly delineates the boundary of the

National Park, abruptly meeting the verdant farmland beneath.

It was with great foresight that the early settlers recognised the vast water-retentive capacity of this mantle of vegetation and protected it as a National Park. It breathes life into the surrounding farms in times of drought. Not all New Zealand forest was spared so assiduously, but much remains. It is possible to walk for days and days in forest wildernesses in New Zealand, something which is only a distant folk memory to those familiar with the highly modified landscapes of Britain.

Away in the far distance, across myriad steep bush-covered ridges, the white summits of the volcanoes in the centre of the North Island gleam as over a sombre sea.

We climbed Mount Taranaki several times. One carefully chosen day in spring we even carried our skis up, and descended that snow-covered scoria in whooping turns. But however much we turned to 'the mountain' for our recreation, we knew we had yet to taste the real promise of this mountain land.

Next summer we were able to take a longer holiday.

We headed to the Southern Alps to see some real mountains. Aotearoa, land of the long white cloud – the Maori name for New Zealand – seems particularly apt for the South Island. Beneath that cloud the shattered brim of the Pacific plate is heaved skywards by tectonic forces as it overrides the Australian plate. These are not the noble stumps of ancient ranges that comprise the Scottish Highlands, but part of a geologically young and active landscape still thrusting up at a steady one inch a year. As we drove south we saw the dramatic wedged peak of Mount Cook (Aoraki, the cloud-piercer), at 12,349 feet, the highest of them all. There he was, glinting – shades and shadows of white – a giant even in the mighty 10,000-foot company of Mount Sefton, La Perouse, Nazomi, Elie de Beaumont and others. This first impact was spectacular and surreal when viewed across the strange turquoise luminosity of Lake Pukaki. (The high content of fine-ground rock or 'glacial flour' in the local lake waters lends them this unusual reflective nature.)

It was Viv's twenty-first birthday. I had given her a wristwatch. I knew it was not enough, that she deserved more from me, but we were still living as penurious students and I knew that she would be offended by more extravagance. Material possessions were relatively unimportant to us: being able to share moments like this, priceless.

We had ten magic days ahead to explore this heartland of the Southern Alps. With growing anticipation we sped the dusty arrow of unsealed road beside the lake. Rapidly the peaks gained stature. We bypassed the small settlement and hotel and pitched our tent at the informal campsite beside an old moraine of the Mueller glacier. Later we rambled to the top in the late afternoon sun, exuberant with the almost palpable aura peculiar to such special places. Even in this sub-alpine zone the biodiversity of fragrant shrubs and herbs was astounding to eyes attuned to the sheep-degraded flora of Britain's wild hills. Mountain flax, snow tussock, snow totara, gaultheria, celmisia (alpine daisies), celery-leaved mountain pine, everlasting daisies, bidi-bidi, raoulia and many others contrived a textured tapestry of intricate form and palette. On the crest we lazed in the warm sun amongst the herbs, and studied the rock and ice of the towering south face of Mount Cook and the stone-strewn glacier grinding towards us from its base.

Isolated huts are dotted far and wide throughout the wilds of New Zealand and we have since spent many nights in their cosy shelter, but our first experience of this New Zealand institution was at the Mueller hut. We reached it after a steep climb from the valley floor sited in a magnificent position at 6000 feet on a ridge opposite the glacier-wreathed, vertical faces of Mount Sefton. A group of fellow trampers sat out in the hot sun, enjoying the spectacle as enormous blocks of ice peeled from precarious positions and cascaded onto the Mueller glacier thousands of feet below. Rather as thunder is heard after the lightning flash, we hunted out the avalanche plumes as sharp cracks and rumbling echoes resounded off rock walls. A family of keas raucously chased scraps of food, the surprising orange of their underwings on take-off a marked contrast to the olive precision of their outer feathers. Far below, on the other side of the ridge, silvery braids of river glinted in the broad waste of shingle stretching from the snout of the Tasman glacier.

Here was geography in the making: terminal, lateral and medial moraines, névés, cirques, truncated spurs, hanging valleys. A living landscape, an alien landscape, but a landscape that had long been in my dreams. I don't think that Frank Smythe ever visited the Southern Alps, but I know he would have been happy there.

Our trip to the Mueller hut was but a short interlude while we waited for an alpine guide to take us on a tour across the Main Divide.

~

Here we were, on the névé of the Franz Josef glacier. The ski plane that had deposited us was a receding buzz. It disappeared over a ridge and the three of us were alone in the centre of a vast silent whiteness. Our guide, Dave, proceeded to initiate us into the intricacies of glacier travel and, as a roped trio, we descended to the Almer hut. The weather was still fine and from our vantage we could see the broken top of the Franz Josef glacier itself. At this point the enormous mass of its névé contorts into the precipitous defile that takes it almost to sea-level on the west coast. The Almer hut perches high on a small rocky island in a sea of ice and snow, yet in sun-warmed rock crevices a beautiful ranunculus displayed its flowers. Who can fail to marvel at the adaptation of seemingly delicate life-forms to such a harsh environment?

We were soon to witness just how harsh it could be. Telltale wisps of cloud from the west presaged a nor'west storm and, in the morning, Dave warned us that we could face difficulties. The alternative of an escape to the west coast down the unstable Franz Josef was not particularly appealing. The weather was still fair, so optimistically we took the risk and set off east for the Graham Saddle.

We ate and packed in a hurry and soon we were muffled in our waterproofs and retracing our steps of the previous day. The pace was fast and the snow quite deep and, although Viv and I were reasonably fit, it was tiring work. The cloud dropped lower until it was only just possible to see nearby rocks through the mist. I was very glad that we were in Dave's expert hands.

As we climbed, the wind increased, the temperature dropped and large flakes of snow began to flail us. Our main concern now was to reach the ridge before conditions became impossible. Viv wrote about the experience from her perspective.

As far as I was concerned conditions were almost impossible now. I could hardly keep up with Dave. The stops to struggle with our crampons and to tie the rope around our waists had frozen my hands and the effort of forcing my tired muscles to move faster seemed to make me colder still. Eventually I felt myself being pulled along by the rope every time I lagged. All the time the wind was whistling bitterly about our faces and visibility was nil.

The ground seemed to come up to meet me and I stopped, only to be jerked by the waist and forced to go on. Instead of having fallen I found I was climbing a near vertical wall of ice-hard snow without a clue as to what was above or beneath. My fear enlivened me and I found new strength to climb. The top of the wall gave onto a level patch of snow and Dave was yelling that we were at the top of the saddle.

Too cold to stop, we pressed on, passed an outcrop of snow-plastered rock and turned into the teeth of the gale. Almost immediately the ground ran away beneath us and we began the descent. Thoroughly heartened I followed, only to come to the lip of a deep, blue-green crevasse and have my newfound courage cut to shreds.

[Little were we to know that the Rudolph Glacier, normally a safe descent, was in Dave's words 'badly cut up this year'. In such conditions it was to be a perilous undertaking.]

We walked along the fissure and found a snow bridge, with no retreat and no other way to cross; I steeled myself and, as the lightest member of the party, crossed first. Keeping my eyes on my feet I tried to walk lightly and fast, while the green depths leered up at me. Safely across I belayed for the others to follow.

Although we were very hungry and lacked energy it was just too cold to stand around, so on we went, crossing smaller crevasses and teetering down rocky ribs on our crampons. Once we had to descend on the path of a stone chute, anxiously looking up in case our passage disturbed a further fall of rocks; and once a descent over rocks was more than I could manage, so the others lowered me down on the end of the rope.

More than once I felt like giving up and sitting in the snow to sleep, but there were always the men, urging me on. Speed was essential. There was still a long way to go.

The clouds seemed to be lifting and the snow becoming lighter and soon we could see down the valley: a waste of moraine, rocks and dirty ice, stretching for miles and miles. In the lee of a huge boulder we fumbled with dates and chocolate although by now I *felt too tired to eat and then, before our muscles seized, we were off again. Now the imminent danger was past, my mind lapsed into semiconscious blankness while my legs and feet marched on... and on.*

With the glowing warmth of the hut, the companionship of its occupants, and a steaming mug of billy tea warming my hands, I began to come out of my fatigued stupor, but it was not until the following morning – Christmas Eve – that I realised how wonderful it was to be alive.

[Our refuge was the de la Bêche Hut. I felt that I too was reaching my limits as we ascended the steep slope of loose moraine to gain that glowing warmth.]

Awakening the next morning I realised the weather had dete-riorated yet again. The wind was muffled and a little snow-light glared through the single windowpane of the bunkroom. I snuggled deeper into the heat of my sleeping bag.

Before long the sound of clumping boots on the wooden floor forced me into an effort to spur myself awake and join John and Dave in their preparations for breakfast.'

All that remained was a misty descent of the Tasman Glacier to the Ball Hut, a welcome bath (a special privilege granted by the guiding company in token of the ordeal we had been through) and a return to our tent the following day.

What sort of man would put his wife through that? We had never planned it that way, but it is what can be expected in the mountains. In better weather we may have danced up the gleaming cones of the Minarets (our planned objective), but fate decreed a darker lesson. After our trip Dave took me aside and told me that Viv was someone very special. He had never seen a woman put up with so much with such courage and no word of complaint. That would be interpreted by some as a sexist remark, but, knowing Viv as I do, it is surely the truth. For three days we had been impressed with the friendly professionalism of this modest man. In true guiding tradition he had put our comfort before his. It was profoundly upsetting to learn of his death in an avalanche a few years later.

In the annals of mountaineering our little adventure would not rate a mention. Joe Simpson, in his remarkable book *Touching the Void*, describes breaking his leg near the summit of a remote

Andean peak, being left for dead after falling into a crevasse, and crawling his way back to base camp to surprise his companions who were sadly and fearfully departing in the sure knowledge of his death. By comparison I have described a stroll over the Graham Saddle in which the participants got a bit wet and tired.

Each to his own threshold of fear and pain, to me the mountains are special: an inspirational package of landform, and natural history – a balm to the soul, a place to share with someone you love. I am in awe of the Whympers, Shiptons, Bonningtons and Simpsons of this world, but for me it is the mountain realm and not the mountaineering that appeals. Physical elevation is less important than elevation of the spirit. We are content to tramp the valleys and passes and merely gaze at the upper heights. A monk at Thyangboche monastery famously remarked to one Himalayan climber, 'Why would I want to tread the snows when I can ascend them in spirit?' A modern answer could be, 'For the adrenalin rush'.

Since the life of a rural veterinarian provides sufficient of these in the normal course of events, as you will see, perhaps I have no need to seek more in times of leisure.

~

'I don't want to be too critical, but why have you reverted to feet and inches for mountains; you who so eagerly advocate the metric system?'

'I did think about that, my dearest. For the practical world of money and science I totally support the logic of metric measures, but for me mountains have always been about dreams, the passion and romance of discovery hidden in dusty tomes. An antiquated system of measurement may be inconsistent with the modern world, but the weight of history is on my side. It suits my purpose. The mountain ranges of the world are arrayed in my mind in feet. I'm sure that Frank Smythe would approve. Let the pragmatists divide my figures by 3.281 if they must.'

CHAPTER TWENTY-ONE

COMMUNICATION IS THE KEY

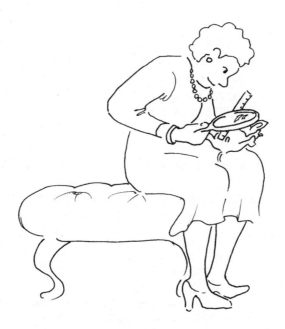

*People don't care how much you know
until they know how much you care.*

For the three years we were in Taranaki we managed to holiday in the South Island at least once a year. There were interesting places to see in the North Island and we visited the volcanic areas, climbed and skied on Ruapehu, but we were forever drawn to the Southern Alps. Although happy in our jobs, I did not want to spend a lifetime as a dairy specialist. I needed to gain experience with other species for which my hard-won years at university had prepared me.

It was time for a change, and a practice in Ashburton on the Canterbury plains was to provide just that. We farewelled our Taranaki friends. Viv forsook her secretarial job for a proofreading one with the local paper, and I forsook dairy cows for a mix of sheep and beef farms, dogs, cats and a smattering of horses. I also came into the sphere of influence of some remarkable vets.

From Kit I learned the value of communication. For Kit, life was for laughs. It is fun to be with such people. He could be careless and made mistakes, as we all do – but he made more than most. A litigious client and clever lawyer could have taken him to pieces. So how did he always come up smelling of roses? Join me in a typical Kit episode.

Mrs Liza Abernethy owned an aggressive little Chihuahua dog called, perhaps, Rastus. Rastus was a type-A personality trapped in a type-Z body. Since life is a matter of mind over matter, and Liza was Z subtype-z, he quite successfully managed to tyrannise his family. I have never been able to understand how such little dogs can hold sway over a group of humans collectively hundreds of times their size, and perhaps intelligence, but it frequently happens. The children in such families often reflect similar behavioural tendencies but, unfortunately, the remedy I am about to describe cannot be applied to them.

Of course the simplistic answer is no longer fashionable. Wild dogs live in a dominance hierarchy. They respect power; the rules of the jungle apply. This doesn't mean that you thrash him every time he growls, although it could well come to the determined and judicious use of a rolled up newspaper, but he certainly should not be accorded preferential treatment. There are psychological ploys to try. He has to be fed as a subservient pack member: after the rest of the family. As with so many pet problems it is the owner who needs the counselling, not the animal. Liza would probably feel so sorry for Rastus that she couldn't bear to see the poor little mite waiting for his food with those big sorrowful eyes. She would persuade herself that her kindness would appeal to his better nature and he would henceforth be a reformed character. Tosh!

In the mid-seventies vets were experimenting with female sex hormones to control aggression in male dogs. It's all so much easier if you can bypass any suggestion of owner inadequacy by providing a solution out of a bottle. Kit had ordered a bottle of slow release progestagen and was itching to experiment. Rastus seemed an ideal subject and was duly injected.

It's quite possible that Kit in his enthusiasm hadn't considered the likelihood of side-effects from his treatment. After all it was only one millilitre that he injected. A small volume, but this was the smallest breed of dog known to man. The one millilitre vial was a standard human female dose. We discussed it amongst ourselves:

'How heavy is Rastus, Kit?'

'About two to three kilos I suppose, Brian.'

'What is the recommended dose for behaviour modification?'

'It's early days; people seem to be a bit hazy about it. Look, do you jokers reckon I've been a bit heavy-handed?'

'Well, the dose you have given him would be sufficient to stop a sixty kilo woman conceiving for six months.'

Kit seemed only slightly fazed. 'When you look at it like that, I suppose it could give his system a bit of a shake up – but at least we'll have given it an honest go and find out if it really works. Besides, I can't very well suck it out again.'

'Yes, but it's going to be a bit expensive treating a Rotty at that sort of dose rate. [Rottweilers are a large breed of dog with a reputation – often misplaced – for aggressiveness.] You could solve China's population problem for marginally less.'

A modicum of disingenuous hyperbole can go a long way. Kit was spurred into action. A few minutes later he was to be seen phoning up pharmacists and the Poisons Centre and doing a rapid literature search focusing on the effects of progestagen overdosage in dogs. Later again he was writing a letter to Liza. The great thing about Kit was that he really did care. The theme of the letter was that he wanted her to record any changes that she noted in the behaviour of Rastus because this was a new technique and any observations would be valuable in helping vets to fine-tune the dosage required. He had just read a very recent paper which said that there might be localised hair loss at the site of the injection and that occasionally the penis could shrink dramatically. Since Rastus wasn't intended for breeding he hoped this wouldn't bother her if it occurred.

Yes, penile atrophy and hair loss were the side-effects of over-dosage. (If someone could market a human drug with exactly the opposite effects they would make a fortune!)

As luck would have it, Kit had chosen a diligent client who entered enthusiastically into the spirit of his inadvert experiment. He received weekly letters from Liza, complete with measurements of Rastus' penile length and he was at great pains to regale us with the details of Rastus' penile regression. This was duly plotted on a 'penis chart' by his desk. The fact that Liza was able to take these measurements was itself testimony to the efficacy of the therapy. No one had even been able to pat his tummy before. Liza was thrilled with the interest and care that Kit had shown for her by now rotund (another side-effect of the progestagen) and contented Rastus. Kit, for his part, was thrilled that Rastus' apparatus stopped shrinking while it still served as a useful conduit for his bladder.

Unfortunately, the causes of aggression in dogs are multifactorial and the solution hardly ever as simple as a single injection. These days there are animal psychologists who make a living attempting to manage such problems. Their approach usually involves adjusting the owners' inconsistencies. A favourable outcome can never be guaranteed so, if children are at risk, and they usually are, there is only one recommendation that I would make. Pets are pets. You should enjoy your relationship; if it has become an ordeal there is something wrong. The unquestioning devotion and playful nature of your dog should comfort, amuse and entertain you and give you good reason for mutually beneficial exercise. If there is any doubt that he might take the face off one of your neighbours' children, he should be euthanased.

~

Most of us carefully conceal areas of knowledge where our professional expertise is thinly spread. But just as the art of good conversation involves a modicum of risk-taking, so the process of acquiring veterinary proficiency necessitates pushing your comfort zones: within reason. As a recent graduate I remember being mortified when an uncle, who happened to be a doctor, asked me a technical question about horse doping, which I couldn't answer.

'But you're a vet now; you're supposed to know about these things.'

Should I have explained that I had spent three years dealing with dairy cows and had hardly touched a horse in that time? That a veterinary degree doesn't teach you everything, but merely provides a foundation on which to build? That you only build on the basis of your interests and experience? I have never had any interest or much contact with the racing industry or doping. Even now, after more than thirty years as a vet, I wouldn't be able to answer his question. No more would he, as a general practitioner, have been able to tell me about brain surgery.

I regret if I have disillusioned those of you who have hitherto had untrammelled faith in our illustrious profession. The fact is no single individual can know everything. The nemesis for many vets is birds. Infrequently they flutter into our lives and, when they do, there is a mad scuffle for textbooks. If the bird is a dead one the scuffle is more leisurely. The usual recourse is to wrap it in plastic and pass the buck to some unfortunate veterinary pathologist at the local animal health laboratory. They then do the autopsy and provide some useful interpretation of their findings that the vet, having clued himself up, can pass back to his client.

Kit had a growing band of admirers. It was amazing to witness the clients who insisted on seeing him; no other vet would do. And Kit was always obliging, always prepared to push the boundaries of his comfort zone. Or perhaps he never knew where they were, but was confident of his supreme ability to talk his way out of uncharted territory. He, however, must have been feeling particularly bullet-proof, or have had an inordinate amount of time on his hands, when he decided to autopsy the budgie himself. This was the budgie that had just died in his hand when he took it off the perch in its cage – unfortunately a not uncommon experience for vets dealing with nervous and sick small birds.

As I recounted to Kit that 'fell off his perch' is a humoristic Liverpool euphemism for death, and 'taken off his perch' didn't have quite the same linguistic resonance, Kit hurriedly explained that he *had* to find something wrong with the wee mite (or words to that effect). He was going to do an autopsy and send anything that looked suspicious to the lab. In due course he found what he took to be abnormal looking lymph nodes in the abdominal cavity and packed them off, all neatly labelled, to the Lincoln Animal Health Laboratory.

All credit to Kit, many vets would have hidden the ensuing report from their colleagues, but we were all allowed to share in what he thought was a huge joke. The report read: 'These were testicles. Birds don't have lymph nodes.'

It would have been interesting to see how Kit explained this to the owner, but in his own consummate style he must have succeeded admirably. The owner came in with his new budgie a short while later for a check-up. 'Is Kit around?'

I felt that it was an enormous privilege to be allowed to learn from another's mistake, and I now see it as a guiding principle in developing a team approach in a veterinary practice. I have little patience with ego-driven prima donnas, derisive of their colleagues. Arrogant attitudes lead to self-delusion and the danger of failing to acknowledge personal mistakes, which is one of the keys to individual growth and learning. There has to be confidence, but there should always be an element of self-doubt. There has to be knowledge, but the ability to communicate it is paramount.

Selecting students for veterinary courses purely on the basis of academic achievement may seem fair, but it does not measure commitment, integrity and character. Nor can it assess the physical aptitudes required for the intricacies of surgery, or the taxing lifestyle of a large-animal vet. These days, such is the demand for places at university veterinary faculties, many young people who would undoubtedly become excellent practitioners fail to achieve the examination requirements for entry. There is far more to being a successful vet than mere academic brilliance.

CHAPTER TWENTY-TWO

LIFE AND DEATH ON THE CANTERBURY PLAINS

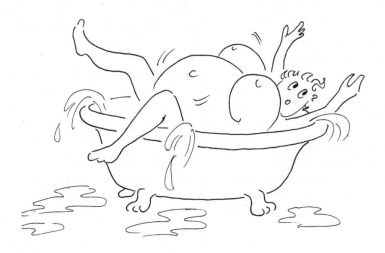

The Canterbury plains, seen from the air, are a neat patchwork of fields and paddocks ranging from rich browns, to greens, greys and yellows depending on the season, and pastoral or arable usage. In the mid-seventies the New Zealand sheep population was around seventy million and the human population about three million – statistics beloved of Australian comedians. Many of these sheep were raised on these plains, ultimately destined for the UK market as Canterbury lamb.

Servicing the sheep industry was a marked contrast to life as a dairy vet. I was happy to meet the new challenge, plus I had the chance to broaden my veterinary skills. Living in a larger town gave me more scope to see pet animals. Working dogs, from sheep and cattle farms, with their broken legs and other injuries gave me a chance to do more surgery. There was also a reasonable amount of horse work, from station hacks to polo horses, from Clydesdales to the Standardbreds used in harness racing. Bud was an equine specialist who performed much of the horse work in the practice.

It takes a quantum leap in approach to deal with the horse-owning public rather than farmers. Showmanship can be important, and an inability to talk the language will mark your inexperience. For the novice vet taciturnity is a good ruse. There is a certain type in the racing industry who can sniff out your cover with ease. Don't say anything!

You espy the stable-hand with the frisky young colt that you are about to castrate. He is a swarthy individual dressed casually in jeans, a dirty shirt and a neckerchief knotted round his throat. Ah! The Romany look. He carelessly chews gum as the colt bounces around beside him on a lead rope. He doesn't deign even to look at you.

'So you're the new vet then.' (Statement. Not a question. No need to reply.) Not replying may be all you need to break the ice. This is not going to be a cordial meeting. You need to assert yourself.

'I'll need a bucket of warm water. If you can fetch that I'll mix up the anaesthetic solution.'

'Bud doesn't use an anaesthetic, he ropes them.'

And he did, it was amazing to witness Bud's tremendous skill at roping down horses. But I wasn't Bud and I was going to have to resort to a conventional anaesthetic. So in this sort of company I said the most appropriate thing.

A grunt followed by, 'OK let's get on with it.'

Welcome to the world of equine practice. Be assertive, take control. Never say 'I don't know'. Substitute a grunt. This is the only exception to my maxim of friendliness and honesty.

Dick Francis would never have been able to make a living writing about sheep farmers, where such flagrant arrogance is extremely rare. It is all so unpleasant and unnecessary. I have never taken a shine to the horse racing industry because of the frequency with which such individuals occur, and so I have had no difficulty following the adage of one of my university lecturers, 'If you are an honest man, don't go into horse practice'. I have to temper this by emphasising that it is a generalisation. I don't wish to tarnish the whole industry, ninety-nine per cent of which gives the rest a bad name.

Equine veterinary practice has taken a long time to catch up with modern ideas but, at the sharp end, money talks and there has been a tremendous amount of research and many impressive advances in recent years. Thirty years ago, a lot of old ideas were fighting a strong rearguard action. The more flamboyant the procedure, the harder it died. Pin-firing injured tendons (where hot needles were passed through to create scar tissue) made as much sense as drilling holes in a steel hawser and filling them with solder to strengthen it; however, it required a major push by the veterinary profession to ban its use by vets who were lured by the showmanship involved. Likewise 'blistering', applying an irritant chemical to the skin over a sprained joint. It worked because it made the leg so sore that the horse was obliged to rest it. Telling the owner to rest his horse for three or four months would achieve the same objective, but lacked the mystery of red blister. Different blisters had their ardent advocates.

At the same time as this mumbo-jumbo was a requisite part of many an equine vet's armoury, the thoroughbred industry forbade the use of artificial insemination to breed foals on the grounds that they would be weaker than foals conceived naturally. Such a ruling would seem to defy common sense, until it is appreciated that the owners of valuable sires had no wish for one ejaculate to inseminate many brood mares, especially when they could command such high fees for natural service. It is interesting to note that the Arabs, with their great tradition of horse breeding, had used artificial insemination techniques – with sponges placed in the vaginas of mated mares and transferred to others – as early as the fourteenth century.

Personally I could never understand the equine practitioner's love affair with stomach-tubes. This involves passing a tube, approximately the width of a garden hose, down a nostril and into the stomach. Great care has to be taken that the tube is not passed down the windpipe, because tipping fluids into the lungs is to pass a death sentence by way of pneumonia. Many horses resent the procedure and usually have to be 'twitched'. With the distraction of a clamp on their nose the tube is passed over the larynx, down the oesophagus and into the stomach.

As a means of generating business it was the tops. Horse-owners felt well satisfied when you had put the worming drench directly into the horse's stomach 'because that's where the bots and worms are'. It seemed patronising to point out that the mouth has a fairly effective connection to the stomach by its own tube. Adding different coloured powders to the mixture, giving it a judicious swirl in the jug and performing the procedure with a practised panache had a certain appeal, but the logic still evades me. I felt that it was intellectually dishonest to promote this practice for routine drenching once worm pastes were widely available, but the idea hung on for years. A farmer could drench thousands of sheep through his yards by mouth, but when it came to his horses they had to be tubed 'to make sure it reaches the stomach'. They wouldn't think of having their children stomach-tubed if *they* had worms. However, good business necessitates keeping the clients happy. Science and business can be uneasy bedfellows.

Myths are not confined to the equine world. Our practice was commissioned to do a trial for a drug company assessing the merits of a new form of bloat prevention in cattle. Bloat is a life-threatening scourge of pasture-fed cattle. For a variety of complex reasons the cow's rumen (stomach) becomes distended with gas to the extent that she is unable to belch it out as she would normally. It presses on the heart and lungs and can quickly lead to death. In severe emergencies stabbing the stomach and letting the gas out through a short tube (trochar) can relieve the internal pressure. The gas is methane and inflammable. Veterinarians with a good sense of timing have been known to light this for dramatic effect, though there are stories of hay barns being burnt to the ground as an unintended side-effect. Holes in cows have to be repaired; a messy job and the cows are often never the same again. Prevention is better than cure.

Drenching twice daily with surfactants, which prevent the formation of foams that cannot be eructated, is an effective preventative used on many dairy farms. It is also practical, because dairy cows come in twice daily for milking. But this is not an option for the beef farmer. On some farms the surfactants can be added to water troughs, but in Canterbury, where much of the farmland is irrigated from a network of water races, that is not practicable either.

The new product was in the form of a palatable block containing the necessary chemicals. The idea was that the cattle obtained enough of the chemical by licking these blocks to prevent bloat deaths. All we had to do was monitor any deaths on the farms chosen for the trial and do post-mortems if necessary to establish the cause of death. After all, in the summer, dead cattle tend to blow up in the sun. Just because she's blown up like a limpet-mine, with legs protruding at weird angles, doesn't mean you can assume that her death was due to bloat. It wasn't always a pleasant job.

When I called in at Trev's place to investigate the dead cow in the middle of his paddock, I couldn't fail to notice a couple of other blown-up carcases partially submerged in the water race.

'Well that one seems to be bloat,' I concluded 'but what about the ones in the water race?'

'Oh they'll just be suckers,' said Trev, rather unhelpfully, although it did look as though he was trying.

'What do you mean?'

'Oh, we've always had those. That's what me old man calls them.'

'Really! But I suspect that they're actually bloat cases that have become incoordinated and then fallen in the water.'

Trev ignored my theory. Generations of cattle must have stumbled into and died in these races, and he wasn't about to relinquish his faith in his father's oft-repeated explanation for my novel ideas. The normal rules of anatomy and physiology, which had hitherto been a useful guide to me, were about to be tested by Trev's more fanciful notions.

'Na, na. They're suckers. See? Their fannies are under water. Once that happens they just suck up the water. They'll be full of water.'

Trev wasn't to be easily convinced, but with a bit of rational debate I could see his lifelong faith in his father's opinion wavering. At times the power of analogy is not to be spurned.

'Look Trev. You're a married man aren't you?'

'Yes.' It was his turn to be puzzled.

'Well, don't you think it would be fair to warn your wife to be very careful next time she has a bath?' He laughed. The light had dawned before I had to prove my point by stabbing the bloated corpses. I wondered if his old man had told him about Father Christmas yet. And then again, had I been the victim of a subtle hoax? If you had met Trev you wouldn't have suggested it. Funny how we can uncritically hold on to long-cherished beliefs. I have done it myself.

CHAPTER TWENTY-THREE

RETURN OF THE NATIVES

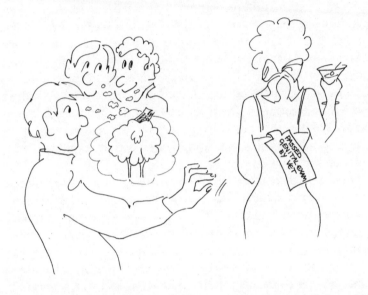

An important element of garden design is to keep the visitor guessing. Straight lines, aside from governing small formal features, are to be avoided. Curves beguile; the whole aspect should never be revealed at a glance. Secret places, surprises, rooms within rooms, are required as part of an intimate plan. Inner landscapes inspire the imagination. This is what the best British landscapes still have to offer, overcrowded though they may be. The Canterbury plains just haven't got it. The pretty patchwork seen from the air is, to all intents and purposes, the whole story. Without the backdrop of the foothills to the Alps it would be soul-destroying. I must add that this is a purely personal observation and most of the inhabitants in the well-kept towns and neat countryside seem to be reasonably sane and happy. The climate, rain-shadowed in the lee of the Southern Alps, is pleasant: sunny and dry much of the time with clear, frosty winter weather. Occasionally nor'west föhn winds blow and these can be hot, dusty and enervating for poor vets wrestling with those rams. Rams without whose services there would be no Canterbury lamb.

The biggest source of veterinary income to the practice during summer was derived from palpating the genitalia of thousands of rams to check they were sound for breeding purposes. New Zealand is unfortunate to have imported the *Brucella ovis* bacterium, perhaps a fair exchange considering other far worse scourges that it fortuitously avoided in its early farming history. *Brucella ovis* prefers to inhabit testicular tissue, where it causes scarring and infertility. By carefully running the testicles through his fingers a vet can feel these lumps. Any affected rams are culled. There is no treatment. The trouble is that by the time the lesions are discernible, the ram is likely to have infected several of his colleagues. Sorry folks, but homosexual activity is a fact of life down on the farm!

These days there is an effective blood test that picks out infected rams at an early stage. If it is used on the rams at a stage of sexual inactivity – at the end of the breeding season – those unfortunates testing positive can be removed before they have a chance to infect their mates. The disease can therefore be eradicated from the flock in a single season, since any ewes infected don't carry the disease from one year to the next. In the mid-seventies this test was in its infancy. So although we were sorting out infected rams, it was but the tip of an iceberg and we were merely slowing the spread of the disease. There were always going to be more to find next year. At the same time as we were feeling for lumps we were also checking for other abnormalities: scrotal hernias, undescended testicles, scrotal mange, pizzle rot and undersized testicles.

As to the latter, size is a relative thing. Since male egos are delicate it doesn't pay to dwell on the statistics too much. Suffice to say, a well-endowed ram can service five- or 600 ewes over a three-week period; although he is usually allotted around a hundred to be on the safe side. If attention is not paid to culling for small testicles, a trait which is inherited, the farmer can eventually end up with rams that can only service fifty ewes. This had happened with some ram breeders who were reluctant to cull fine-looking rams on the basis of testicular size. And here we should leave any unsavoury parallels between ovine and human reproductive capacity, but perhaps we won't.

A farm with 2000 ewes could have twenty to forty rams. There is no point putting unsound rams with your ewes to compete with the fertile ones. They need to be rooted out by those perspiring vets. Watch them as they crouch in that race full of rams. Each ram's genitalia is palpated for defects. Crouch, palpate the two or three rams within arms' reach; stand, wade past them and find space to crouch again. Repeat, repeat, repeat. If there is space behind you with only one or two rams, be aware! They are not at their most cooperative as the breeding season advances and testosterone pervades their minds and bodies. Their testicles become more turgid. The skin in the groin becomes flushed. Is this the origin of the expression 'in the pink'? Alas my dictionary of etymology would not have it so. It must be wrong. What of 'pizzle rot', then? Surely that is not also an allusion from *Romeo and Juliet*? Thank goodness not. Shakespeare had no hand in it. There is no romance in pizzle rot for this is 'characterised by ulcerative lesions with scab formation on the prepuce', usually predisposed by rams producing alkaline urine from a high protein diet. This damages the delicate mucous membrane lining, allowing a bacterial infection to supervene. There, I just thought you'd like to know in case it crops up in *Trivial Pursuit*.

If the rams were from a ram breeder and going to a sale, a metal clip was attached to the wool. In distinctive white writing on a red background it stated 'passed genital examination by a vet'. The shearers didn't like these because if they weren't removed after the sale they could damage their finely tuned gear. The clips were soon phased out, but they retained some value amongst the party set.

One farm completed, on to the next. It could be hard work, more a challenge than a problem for a fit young vet. I enjoyed it. Meanwhile there was the opportunity to see different farming systems and interact with the fascinating array of types that comprise the New Zealand farmer. The large-animal practitioner is fortunate to have a percentage of his time occupied by relatively mindless tasks, time to retreat into mental relaxation, make small talk, and contemplate the inadequacies of his genitalia. Small-animal practice may be less physically demanding, but there is no mental let-up, as I was soon to find out.

Viv's job as a proofreader was not particularly inspiring. We found it quite difficult to find time to escape into the hills. We were childless when we no longer wanted to be. I had gained valuable experience in this job, but it was time for a change.

Like many immigrants we had taken that fateful mid-winter holiday. Winging back to England in late spring, seeing those hedgerows frothing into life, catching up with loved ones. Balmy outings through hazy sunlit landscapes. Yes! We hit one of those vintage summers: visits to ruined abbeys, stately homes. Holiday time, relaxation, no work, no after-hours calls: rose-tinted spectacles. We responded to a five-year itch and decided to return to England. We thought it would be for good.

CHAPTER TWENTY-FOUR

TOY REPAIR MAN

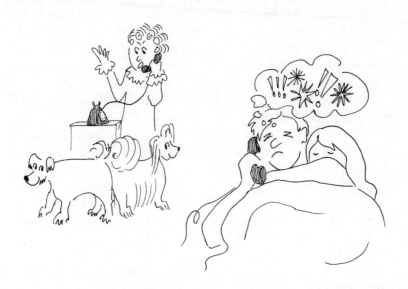

The New Zealand Veterinary Club system was a remarkable institution. Groups of farmers had banded together throughout the country, each with the purpose of attracting vets to service farms in their area. The first New Zealand graduates didn't escape the doors of Massey University till 1971, and there was still a deficit out in the field for several years after. To fill the gap the Veterinary Services Council (VSC) had been set up which actively helped vets from overseas, such as me, to immigrate. They also laid down standard terms of service and award-rates which applied uniformly across the country to all vets working in 'vet clubs'. It was a model system, and it discouraged the rampant exploitation of young vets that is so prevalent in Britain. For older vets it did have its drawbacks and the system has all but folded, but it served its purpose well, and most rural New Zealand townships now have a thriving veterinary clinic. When the club system was strong and vets were scarce private practices in New Zealand were obliged to compete with the clubs and employ vets on favourable terms.

On our return to England, by contrast, I was about to find out what unthinking capitalism can do. The theory is to climb the ladder as fast as possible so that you are in a position to exploit the next generation of new graduates, as you yourself have been exploited. The suicide rate in vets in Britain is higher than for any other profession, mostly in younger vets who are unable to match their high expectations with the reality of the daily and, all too frequently, nightly grind.

There was no shortage of jobs. I had excellent references and we had a good poke around various parts of England looking for a job in a mixed practice. Salaries for veterinary assistants were, however, abysmal. At that stage British lorry drivers were on strike for an increased pay award. I recall that they were already earning more than most of the practice principals were prepared to offer a vet with five years' experience. I have no wish to detract from *their* claim, but most veterinary positions then committed you to a ten- to twelve-hour day followed by a one-in-two to one-in-six (depending on the size of the practice) roster for weekends and night duty. It was preferred that you were married and that your wife would be around, unpaid, to answer the phone if you were out when on duty. These terms were usually accepted without question, all part of the privilege of being a vet, but Viv and I drew the line at the flat above the clinic. The flat where you would be on duty even when you were not on duty, prey to any passing member of the public who noticed the vet sign and decided to drop in at any time of the day or night.

Eventually we decided on a predominantly small-animal practice in Yorkshire, in a semi-rural area immediately adjacent to Ilkley Moor – as immortalised in that ghastly folk song. The moor itself is a grim polluted upland, soured by acid rain and blackened by decades of soot from the hundreds of square miles of factory and domestic chimneys in the large towns swarming its southern edge. But this is a point of demarcation, to the north and west there is open country, a corridor to the less crowded fells and dales. Away to the east are the wonders of York, a city full of incredible historical and architectural associations; a place to which we still readily return.

Craig, the practice principal, was an extremely progressive veterinarian. Not only did he offer me a reasonable salary, but also – the main appeal – the opportunity to develop another set of professional skills. There were only three of us, so it was down to a one-in-three roster. I failed to realise that this would practically guarantee that I would be called from my bed every third night. Shift workers returning from their jobs in the dark, satanic mills of Leeds and Bradford were not averse to phoning at two or three in the morning because they had found 'brown things crawling' on their dog, a fair description of fleas. Once you have swum and clawed your way to the surface of consciousness from the depths of sleep deprivation to respond to a question like that, it is extremely difficult to relax again.

The vet's hours on duty are never in shifts. The vet who finishes his evening surgery at 7.25 pm, attends a pony with colic at 9.00 pm (with the expectation that he will be back to it again in the middle of the night) and performs a caesarean on a bitch at 4.00 am, is the same one who fronts up at 8.30 am for the start of another day. For the salaried vet there is no extra remuneration for the inconvenience. It has always been regarded as part-and-parcel of the job. No vet objects to a genuine emergency call out, but it is fielding the trivia from the inconsiderate that really grates. One tends to have an uncharitable disposition on such occasions.

And now gentle reader, avid consumer of all those vet books, I will let you into a little secret: the results of a survey I have conducted amongst my colleagues. We are not all angels. When we tumble from our beds and get into our cars to attend your dog/cat/horse/cow we do not always think, 'How blessed am I, for I have been presented with the opportunity to alleviate great pain and suffering'. Or even, 'How selfish of me to have that pang of resentment. I will have to miss our Johnny's prize-giving because it's my duty to attend to Mr Pain-in-the-Arse's constipated dog, which has been off colour for a week, but is in desperate need of attention NOW'.

No, sad to relate, most of us (with the exception of James Herriot and Sinatra), sit in the car and, in New Zealand parlance, 'throw a wobbly' – scream, swear, maybe both. If we are really tired and haven't the youth or energy for such hysterics, a depressed resignation assails our souls. Rest assured your veterinarian will, having let off the requisite amount of steam, attend your pet with full professional dignity in the former instance, and with monosyllabic competence in the latter.

Occasionally from the warmth of our beds we will try and defer requests in order to attend animals at more civilised hours. Some requests are for advice only. The story is told of the client who rang her vet around bedtime because her dog had 'got stuck to' her neighbour's bitch. For anyone who knows about dogs and dog breeding, or has been brought up on the mongrel-strewn streets of Liverpool, this would obviously be recognised as a classic case of 'tying'. During mating, a swelling at the base of the dog's penis effectively locks into the vagina of the bitch preventing a dignified dismount and withdrawal. After dismounting the dog is still linked to his heart's desire. The very act of dismounting puts the two of them back to back.

Although this might appeal to the lyricists of country and western music, our two canine lovers have, by contrast, had a satisfying tryst and are now 'tied' like a 'push-me-pull-you' shunting train. It can take fifteen or twenty minutes for the dog's tumescent penis to subside sufficiently for the pair to separate. How the course of history would have been altered if mankind were similarly endowed. Instances of couples caught *in flagrante delicto* would be common place. The whole pace and thrust of bedroom farces would be changed.

When Mrs Innocentia phones Barry Hardcastle, her long-suffering vet, he explains to her briefly that what is occurring is perfectly normal and that if she waits a little while all will be well. Perhaps he should have explained things a bit more fully, but, as you shall see, he had other things on his mind. Ten minutes later the phone rings again.

'I'm sorry to bother you again Mr Hardcastle, but Roger's still stuck to Virginia.' There is a pause at the end of the line, as Barry's mind is required to make a quantum leap back into the real world.

'I'll tell you what, Mrs Innocentia. You put the phone down now and when I ring back put me onto Roger.'

'I don't see how that's going to help.'

'Well it's just worked for me!'

If you want to get the best out of your vet my recommendation is to lie. Psychologists have determined that even the most honest of us lie around a hundred times a day, perhaps starting with 'Good morning'. It's amazing how incredibly helpful it is if that midnight request is prefaced with, 'I'm terribly sorry to bother you, but…'. Lies in these instances are important social lubricants. Civilisation would disintegrate without them. The person who interrupts your sleep with a blunt 'I've got a dog I want you to look at' is at grave risk of adding to his bill unless he is subsequently appreciative of your sacrifice, or due allowance can be made for his loss of manners owing to the stress of a genuine emergency. It therefore literally pays to be polite, in my book anyway. Being assertive is all very well, but I do try to do my part in ensuring that the meek shall inherit the earth.

Vets have to balance conflicting moral pressures. The difference in approach required by farm-animal and small-animal clinicians is a prime example. A cynic once distilled this into a simple philosophy: as a farm vet you are helping your clients to make more money, in small-animal practice you are a toy repair man. In mixed practice you may at one minute sacrifice a sick lamb to establish the cause of a problem afflicting a flock, and the next you are using refined surgical techniques on a budgie to remove a tumour. I think the only common thread is that in either instance the task is undertaken humanely. Economics do ultimately govern all farm-animal decisions, and the owners' wishes all pet-animal work. How is it otherwise possible to rationalise cutting a sick lamb's throat at 4.00 pm, yet splinting a sparrow's broken leg at 5.00 pm? For most of us the interest and variety inherent in a veterinary career more than compensate for the burden of such philosophical dilemmas.

CHAPTER TWENTY-FIVE

IMAGE IS EVERYTHING

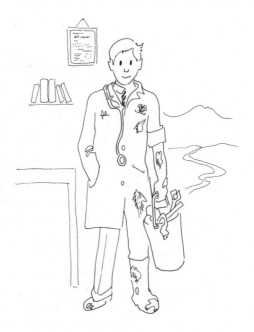

Perhaps I had spent too long in the colonies and acquired bad habits, but it wasn't long before Craig suggested that I wore a suit to work. A sports jacket and tie would be acceptable in large-animal practice, but he felt that presenting the right image to the public was paramount. In general I agree that cleanliness and tidiness are virtues, but wearing a suit seemed a bit over the top. I still had the suit I had purchased for my university interviews and I was not prepared to buy another. Accidents happen in vet clinics and emptying the impacted anal glands of a dog in a new suit smacked of overkill.

This image thing was taken very seriously. One of the neighbouring practitioners had decorated the walls of his waiting room with thoughtfully posed photographs of himself in a white coat with a stethoscope draped casually around his neck. I was perhaps lucky that Craig did not hold the same proclivity towards showmanship. We donned snazzy blue dentist tops for our consultations, leaving the trousers exposed to any animal detritus that projects, weeps, exudes, discharges or splashes. It was therefore more practical if these were of dark colours, and we relied on the human nose being a thousand times less sensitive than its canine equivalent.

Behind the scenes, standards were high. Craig employed qualified animal nurses and the latest equipment – ultrasonic dental scalers, electrocautery and an early blood analyser – so that we could get quick results rather than sending samples to a laboratory. Yet, at this time, some British practices didn't even have a basic anaesthetic machine. I was pleased to be in a progressive practice, and I certainly gained valuable experience in the eighteen months that I worked there. I did not resent fitting in with the cultural ethos of the practice and indeed was happy to make readjustments to other colonial transgressions I may have been making. I quickly discovered that these were not merely sartorial. I required some social re-engineering.

I had been educated in a school where all boys were addressed by surname only.

'Hoffman! Can you tell me whether the word "orange" in this sentence is a verb or a noun?' Big pause – during which a clearly confused Hoffman, after a series of erratic answers, faces the terror of a caning if he gets this one wrong.

'You haven't done your homework, have you boy?' Pause. 'Well is it a "doing" word?'

Hoffman falls into the trap with a tentative, 'Yes, sir.'

'Very well Hoffman, come to the front of the class and show us all how to "orange".'

Hoffman deliberates. 'I can't, sir.'

'All right, Hoffman. Report to me at the end of class.'

We very quickly discovered how to learn from others' mistakes. But sometimes we were pushed too hard. It was the same long-suffering Hoffman, an unathletic boy, who inadvertently managed to extract some revenge on a Physical Education teacher. With great effort he had climbed the bars in the gymnasium and hung alongside others of us who had attained the same position by climbing the ropes. We had been made to hang from the top bar about five metres off the floor while Hoffman lumbered up. He wasn't exactly popular with us either, but 'Mong', a master with distinctly Sinaean features (and woe betide he caught you using his nickname), thought that Hoffman could do with a taste of what we were enduring. He casually paced up and down below us, detailing ever so slowly and deliberately what we were to do when we had climbed back down the ropes. Hoffman, even though he had only recently joined our elevated position, seemed to be suffering more than the rest of us.

'Please, sir, I'm going to fall.'

'Don't worry, Hoffman, your sense of self-preservation is too strong. Now...' His leisurely dissertation was interrupted by a thud as Hoffers hit the deck. There was subsequently an enquiry into Hoffman's broken ankle. It seemed no coincidence that Mong left soon afterwards and plagued us no more. Rumour had it that he became a sheep farmer in New Zealand. I have yet to meet him in Godzone.

On leaving school in Britain your surname is dignified by a respectful 'Mr'. Imagine the relief this would have accorded the likes of Mr Hoffman as he departed the school gates for the last time. It would have been gratuitous to use Christian names. To be on 'Christian name terms' with someone was a status earned after close bonding and almost exclusively amongst friends, or by used-car salesmen shamefully unaware of social boundaries. After all, we were not that distant from Dickensian days when some spouses addressed even each other as 'Mr' and 'Mrs'. How strange to find a New Zealand where murderers and politicians enjoyed the sweet privilege of first name status and everyone seemed to be on first name terms. But New Zealand is manifestly a more friendly society. Brits are definitely more reserved. There are pros and cons. Who wants to be tricked into feeling warm fuzzies about their Minister of Finance? On the other hand, relationships in the workplace are more relaxed if the boundaries are less formal.

Returning to the land of my birth it now felt distinctly odd to be addressed as 'Mr Hicks' by the nurses, although I could use *their* first names. The rules of an invisible hierarchy were rigidly upheld. I could address my veterinary colleagues by their Christian names in their presence, but in front of clients or the nurses I had to refer to them by surname.

All in all it took a while to adjust back to life in Britain, and it wasn't just socially. We had selected an area where we could indulge in the England of our dreams. We were within an hour or two of our families, beautiful dales, wild fells and the ancient city of York. We had purchased a house. We intended to settle and make a go of our new life, but after a few months it was apparent that New Zealand had altered our horizons and expectations. Time and again I would return from my evening clinic mentally exhausted. My job was interesting, but demanding. I didn't have the energy after a week at work to face the traffic jams and drive to York. We visited our parents, but it is always a mistake to think that you can revisit your childhood. The relationship between independent, adult children and their parents should rightly be that of a respectful and loving friendship. Distance cannot dim it if the channels of communication are maintained, and in our case they have been. The glories of the English countryside are undeniable, but we had also experienced and grown to appreciate something else.

As far as my work was concerned I found myself increasingly out of sympathy with my role as a toy repair man. Treating the family pet is one thing, but small-animal veterinarians have to deal frequently with animal hobbyists, be they cat fanciers or dog breeders, and I must admit to being a trifle unnerved by some of their obsessions. The further we move from the original working purpose of the animals in our lives, the more unbalanced we become in our attitudes towards them. Vets frequently have to deal with raving nutcases; those people you read about with seventeen cats in their houses are not uncommon. The mentality behind breeding animals with gross anatomical deformities for the novelty of their appearance and then devoting your weekends to primping them up and exhibiting them at shows also disconcerts me. Look objectively at the surgical and medical interventions required to keep some of these monstrosities alive in a world where such resources are in short supply, even for humanity. To my mind these are manifestations of a sick society. I was out of sympathy with FruFru ('not like that, there is a hyphen between "Fru" and "Fru"'), mincing along the city pavement with his poodle trim and tartan coat. I wanted to get back to the real dogs: Fleur, Jake, Rak, Wag, Gin, Tug, Dart, Teak, Sky. Dogs that have a respectful working bond with their shepherds. Dogs eager, even joyful, at their work, as they drive streams of mustered sheep from their rocky ridges and through the tawny tussock.

It wasn't easy to tell our families for a second time that we were emigrating to New Zealand, but the prospect of life as a veterinary practitioner in Britain filled me with dread. The image is not the reality.

I reiterate: the suicide rate for vets in Britain is higher than in any other profession.

CHAPTER TWENTY-SIX

DEAR DEER

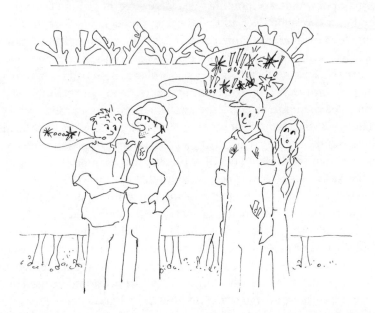

By the late 1970s the New Zealand economy was starting to suffer. There had been years of steady prices for agricultural produce due to a dependable trade with the parent country. Alas, Britain now saw its future in Europe and the Common Market. It was difficult for New Zealand to adjust after withdrawal of the benefits that the previous trading relationship with Britain had conferred on all its citizens: the days when it had, per capita, one of the highest standards of living in the world.

The New Zealand to which Viv and I returned was entering a recession. One consequence for us was that there were very few veterinary jobs available. Our hearts were sold on the South Island, but it looked as though – horror of horrors – we would have to go to Southland. The rest of New Zealand regards this province as a cold, wet wasteland. Next stop Antarctica.

With few other options open to us we decided that I should take up a six-week locum position in a vet club in Western Southland. At least the discomfort would only be temporary.

With depressed prices for meat and wool, farmers were looking at alternatives to traditional sheep farming. Deer farming held promise and enterprising individuals were laying the foundations of a major new industry. Southlanders were in at the ground floor, they had access to wild deer and wild entrepreneurs. The former came courtesy of liberations of red deer into the bush and mountains nearly a hundred years earlier. There were even their larger cousins, North American Elk, released into Fiordland. Both had been hunted by generations of vigorous Southlanders, many of them farmers, many of them attracted to the challenge of farming their quarry. There was the glamour of looking out of the window of your farm-house and watching them drift past. These new devotees tended to look down on those who still chose to farm 'ground lice', though personally I would never be so disparaging as to use this expression to describe sheep grazing at pasture. It cannot be denied that the New Zealand economy has grown on the sheep's back.

For vets it was also a new challenge. Wild animals were being bulldogged or net-gunned out of helicopters, darted with drugs, or even physically manhandled out of home-made traps at the edge of the bush and released onto farms. What drugs should be used and at what dose rates? How do you physically handle these powerful animals? What animal health problems are likely to occur and how do we deal with them? Answers to these questions came mostly empirically – it was largely a matter of trial and error.

Deer, for instance, when running in a mob, will keep to the edges of a race leading into a shed. Cattle in similar situations run down the centre. If a mob of cattle runs towards you in a raceway, step to one side and they will rush past you. Witness the laggards at Pamplona during the running of the bulls. Because deer hug the fences, it is better to stand in the centre if caught in such circumstances and let them mêlée past on either side. The odd one may take the shorter route over the top of you, but it beats getting rolled along the netting by a mob of panicking hinds or stags. Yards were being designed to work with deer psychology to minimise handling, especially with the larger elk-type deer. These had hybridised with red deer in the wild and the mix, generally designated Wapiti (an Indian name for elk), are large and often ill-tempered. No matter, in these heady early days there was a shortage of deer for farming and anything resembling a deer was worth a lot of money. Dealers weren't going to cull a $5000 hind merely because she tried to kill anyone who got in the yards with her. It was a case of *caveat emptor*. Such animals tended to be sold on to another poor unfortunate.

It was soon evident that deer are susceptible to tuberculosis and the biggest task for vets involved with the deer industry was to keep up with the TB-testing. This involved clipping hair off the neck with noisy clippers at the end of a long flex, not easy in a pen of milling deer, and then injecting a small dose of tuberculin into the skin. In the early days, particularly, when selection of animals for good temperament was secondary to building up numbers, and facilities were inadequate, this could be a time-consuming and demanding job. I likened it to one memorable description of warfare – *long periods of boredom punctuated by brief moments of terror.*

A crash helmet of some sort was advisable because deer tend to attack by standing on their hind legs and striking down on the head with their front feet. Some heroes disdained such protection but, if they commented on my routine of donning my trusty cricket helmet, I took pleasure in explaining that some people have thicker skulls than others. Footwear is also important. Gumboots used by foresters offer chainsaw protection, ideal against the sharp pointed hooves of deer. Standard gumboots are about as useful as condoms when a 200-kilo stag decides to pirouette on your toe.

With the Marshall brothers there was less danger. You could always rely on them putting their burly bodies on the line first. It was a pleasure to work with such a team, despite an atmosphere invariably replete with invective.

As a veterinary practice we willingly hosted young students eager to discover if vetting was the vocation for them, just as I had as a teenager with Mr Betts. One morning a particularly demure young lady accompanied me as we set off to develvet some stags for the Marshalls. As we drove up to the shed I warned her about the language she would encounter.

As we got out of the car we could hear the anticipated encouragement the boys inside were giving their stags as they sorted them into pens, from the relatively mild 'now get in there you fat bastard' to 'grind your f***ing teeth at me one more time, you c*** , and I'll cut your bleeding head off'. We waited outside till the sorting was done. Soon the banging of doors and swearing stopped and one of the brothers emerged sweating but satisfied.

'Gidday, John. Roughly forty of the bastards to do today. We've put some in the new pens on the outside. We can do those c**** first.' He then noticed the girl following behind me and demonstrated that even the Marshall brothers had chivalric boundaries.

'You might have f***ing warned me, you bastard!' he growled.

Develvetting is a misunderstood procedure and was banned in Britain on humanitarian grounds under the mistaken belief that it involved stripping the velvet skin off the antlers which develop each spring. In fact the entire antler is removed before it hardens, and in a way which is more reliably humane than the similar procedure of dehorning cattle. Furthermore, without antlers stags are less dangerous to their handlers and other animals.

The technique used on the Marshalls' farm, where they didn't have a crush to hold the stags, involved going around a set of smallish pens, where they had been sorted approximately four to a pen, and injecting each with a sedative. By the time the stags in the last pen were injected, those in the first were dopey enough to be approached to give a local anaesthetic nerve block. When each had received his nerve block, it was time to start at the beginning again and saw off the antlers. Mature stags can yield several kilos of velvet and, at a price of over a hundred dollars a kilo, it was a valuable product.

Of course events don't always run so smoothly. The odd stag required a heavier dose of sedative and would need to be re-injected. Particularly flighty animals could get jumpy and damage the velvet of others in the same pen. There was usually something to keep the adrenalin flowing.

The Marshalls' new pens were rather makeshift. The walls were made from sheets of plywood. They came down to near floor level with a gap underneath. As we came back to the first pen to saw off the velvet the stags were resting peacefully, but a couple of them had an antler through the gap. No problem. We rolled the first into a sitting position. Funny! It was easier than expected. Any velvet protruding beyond the pen had been removed. Same with the next stag. At least the analgesia had worked well. Those two stags had lain motionless while a few hundred dollars worth of velvet was gnawed off their heads. A rather pleased-but-anxious-looking dog could be seen on the other side of a gate. The tip of his tail wagged, in a gesture of appeasing enquiry. Soon he was a mere speck in the distance, blasted there by gales of unrepeatable invective. He still looked fit and healthy at my next visit when I remarked on his shiny coat and enquired what they could have been feeding him...

Velvet is widely used in Eastern medicine and not merely as an aphrodisiac, as is widely supposed. Deer farmers who have been overseas and witnessed deer farming and velvet harvesting in Korea and China report that the spilt blood was collected and drunk on the spot. I had the opportunity to wipe the saw I used for develvetting, so once, and to my regret, I decided to try a little taster. It repeated on me for the rest of the day. The farmer with me declined graciously, 'Any more and I'd be dangerous!'

Deer pizzles are another valuable by-product of deer farming, and also used in Eastern medicine. Unfortunately, harvesting these is a terminal, rather than an annual, event.

~

Jim Kane was more interested in deer capture than farming. An experienced pilot, he had survived a few chopper prangs, although sadly a fatal one was waiting to claim him before the year was out. Jim installed a manager on his farm while he pursued his vocation – capturing the biggest Wapitis he could out of the Fiordland bush. These were large, mean and valuable. A Wapiti stag could be worth $10,000. This figure is etched in my mind.

It is daunting stepping into a pen with animals of this size. Being able to look down on a stag confers a definite psychological advantage. It cuts both ways. Stags respect size too. You have to look up to mature Wapiti stags. But life as a deer vet was becoming a little easier since we adopted pole syringes. These enabled us to keep a metre or so from the animal we were injecting.

And there I was, sedating stags that a few weeks earlier had been free agents in the mountain forests of Fiordland. They didn't seem to appreciate the promise of a carefree existence as a sire stag on a farm, and weren't about to relinquish their velvet to me gracefully. The largest one – 'Look at this one John, Jimmy caught him last month. He reckons he's worth at least ten grand' – was particularly fired-up and grinding his teeth aggressively. I gave him the standard dose of sedative. When we came back to the pen it was as though nothing had happened. Ten-Grand was unimpressed with my style of chemical warfare. His chemical, adrenalin, was stronger than mine. Nothing for it, I felt, but to repeat the dose. We continued with our routine. When we got back to the pen ten minutes later Ten-Grand was dead. Soon after we heard the throb of a helicopter as Jim flew over and dropped in to review proceedings. There was nowhere to hide.

Jim looked at what had been his $10,000 and at the man who had indirectly prevented him from banking it. It was hard telling him what had happened.

'No problems, John. These things happen when you're working with deer.' True Jim, but it takes great generosity of spirit to contemplate such a loss without a trace of anger or blame.

Such accidents are an occasional and inevitable consequence of working with semi-wild animals. Nobody feels good about them, but every vet will have to face similar experiences at some stage in their careers. How they cope will, to a large extent, depend on the attitude of the owner with whom they are dealing and, especially if they are a young vet, the support they receive from their colleagues.

Furthermore, the presently evolving environment of blame supported by litigation needs to be carefully balanced. In the long run, aside from blatant cases of professional negligence or incompetence, litigation is not in the best interests of the majority of the animal-owning public. Funds to pay for the ever-increasing cost of professional indemnity insurance ultimately have to be financed through more expensive vet fees, or withdrawal of services that have been identified as being at high risk of litigious claims, whether justified or not. This has already happened in some areas of equine medicine, a high risk area for vets.

CHAPTER TWENTY-SEVEN

LITANY AND LITIGATION

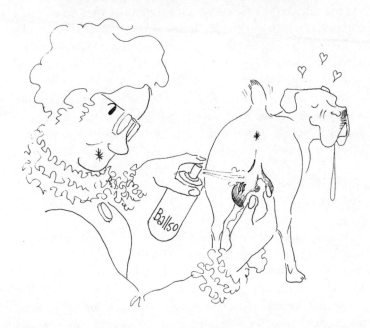

Most of the vets I have worked with have been conscientious almost to a fault. Their neglected families will testify to this. At all times they genuinely strive to do their best for their patients. Sometimes it isn't good enough. Mistakes are made. The first important step is to acknowledge them. A culture of blame and heavy litigation prevents that first step happening. Any insurance policy advises the insured not to accept liability even if he is sure that the mistake is attributable to his negligence.

I have never faced litigation myself but, seeing innocent colleagues keel-hauled through the court system, I have always felt there to be an element of, 'There but for the grace of God go I'.

Soon after the Ten-Grand episode I was called, once again, to examine my shortcomings and write one of the most difficult letters of my life:

Dear Sarah

This is a hard letter for me to write, but not as hard as the upset that you will have been through since the sad loss of Bobby.

What happened was an accident and I hope you can understand that. Despite the best will in the world, they do and will happen. That doesn't make it any easier to accept when the consequences are the loss of a much-loved pet and I know that if the same thing happened to our own little dog I would also be deeply upset.

Whilst nothing can replace Bobby, or compensate for the hurt you must feel, I have come to an arrangement with your father which may help a little bit. In time I hope that you can accept my sincerest apologies for my part in your loss.

Yours sincerely
John Hicks

It was my fault. When I had returned to the clinic from castrating a colt, I hadn't re-labelled a bottle of unused anaesthetic solution as ten per cent strength and a colleague had unknowingly taken it off the shelf assuming that it was the usual five per cent. Bobby died of an anaesthetic overdose given for a routine operation.

Explaining this to a little girl is about as tough as it gets, but Sarah's father, although upset, was understanding and fair. The compensation mentioned allowed him to purchase another Cairn Terrier puppy for his daughter. He sought no more than that. If the claim had been higher I would have been resorting to our insurance protection scheme. Technically I could have been sued for professional negligence.

~

In the USA storm clouds of litigation loom over vets in the same manner as those (often apocryphal) stories about the American medical profession. Vets in practice in the States can even donate to bogus animal welfare societies. These act as fronts whose main function is to dissuade potential litigants from prosecuting. Excessive litigation leads to corruption.

It may seem an unrelated fact, but also in the States there is a company that manufactures artificial testicles to replace those removed from your pet dog during castration. One of the benefits promoted for their use being to help your animal's self-esteem. Your neutered pet can then roll on his back in front of visitors, without shame, and flaunt prosthetic testicles of appropriate (or inappropriate) size. Different textures are available ('natural' or 'original') should your guest feel the need to fondle them. You may also be surprised to learn that the company markets key-rings, tote bags and t-shirts promoting these farcical products.

Neutered dogs are not usually permitted in the show ring, so there has been some consternation in show circuits round the world.

Dear Mrs Gropenuts

We are disappointed to learn of your decision to sue Dr Rinkle-Sachs following a surgical misadventure that occurred when he was implanting testicular prostheses into your Boxer dog, Conker.

He was deeply contrite to learn that the scars are clearly visible after you have cleaned and polished Conker's scrotum and that this has severely compromised Conker's chances of competing successfully on the dog show circuit.

You may not be aware, but Dr Rinkle-Sachs has been a life-long supporter of the Bollocksville Animal Lovers Liberation Society (Inc), BALLS, a registered charitable organisation. Without his regular and generous contributions we will find it hard to continue our work of capturing testicularly compro-mised stray dogs and restoring them to visually acceptable testicular normalcy and preventing the complex of psychoses that might otherwise result in euthanatization [sic].

We would ask you to re-consider your claim for $100,000 damages, including damages for anticipated loss of prize money from showing/displaying Conker and loss of tactile pleasure incurred from polishing Conker's scrotum, and reflect instead on the effect this will have on the distinguished career of Dr Rinkle-Sachs.

If your litigation succeeds there is a risk that Dr Rinkle-Sachs will develop behavioural aversion (testicular) syndrome (BATS). An independent psychiatric assessment from Dr Priapus has warned us that this could result in institutionalization.

We ask you to take these factors into consideration before proceeding with your suit.

Yours truly
Orchitis Wrangler Jnr

Don't look at me like that! Alright, perhaps the letter is fictitious, but I can imagine Mr Bett's eyebrows twitching at the strange ethical switches required of a profession which is no longer an arbiter of animal welfare. If we follow the American model, it seems, our standards must follow the dictates of the marketplace. Then we shall achieve financially; its sole criterion of success.

CHAPTER TWENTY-EIGHT

HOLIDAY IN HOSPITAL

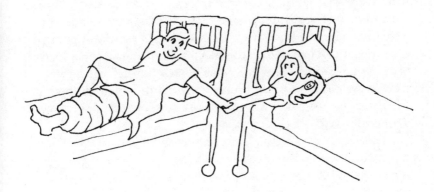

The head of the hatchet was firmly wedged in the block of firewood that I was attempting to split. In an attempt to free it, I belted it with a hammer. Fateful mistake, John! A shard of steel shot out from the impact with the velocity of a bullet and into my tensed thigh. Look! It's frayed the fabric of my trousers. Hardly a mark on my skin, though and yet... yes, my leg is starting to feel tight.

I imagined this tiny fragment shearing through the fibres of my quadriceps and severing some deep-seated blood vessel. That is precisely what had happened. An x-ray revealed the culprit had traversed several inches of flesh and was nestling next to my thigh bone (femur).

This wasn't very good timing. Emily was just over two years old and our new baby was due any moment. I had had the skill-saw 'surgery' on my finger immediately before Emily's birth, and it had provided a sound test of our resource-management skills. I suspected that Viv wasn't going to be too impressed with the prospect of a repeat performance. We were new to the district and, like many immigrants, we had no family support in place should things go wrong.

My blood pressure was sky high.

Surgery couldn't be delayed. We had no choice. Almost the next thing I knew, I was recovering from what I presumed would have been fairly routine surgery. It was night, but as an older generation would say, that leg was giving me 'gyp'. Trying to find a small piece of metal buried in the largest muscle mass in the body must have been a bit like hunting for a needle in a haystack, so perhaps the surgeon had had to dig around a bit. But the pain should have been easing, not increasing. Moans floated through the darkness from other beds, pit-patter scurrying, curtain-drawn-whispering. They were busy. I didn't want to make a fuss, but the plea escaped my lips. Nurse!

Analgesia has its limits. Despite the nursing staff reluctantly dispensing ever more powerful pain-killers I was now in a drugged state of agony. A tighter bandage was put round my thigh, and then a tighter one. That is a night I shall never forget.

When I woke up I was lying in a considerable amount of blood. As an aspiring vet student it had taken a fair amount of objectivity to learn to be unfazed by the sight of blood, and indeed I was: as long as it was not my own. Suddenly the body language of the hospital staff implied hurried professionalism. They were dealing with a serious haemorrhage. In the light of day I must have appeared very pale, a blood test showed that my red cell count had dropped alarmingly. It was too low for them to risk giving me a full anaesthetic, but they had to stop that bleeder soon. So a sweating junior doctor probed deeply into my leg. He was (desperately) trying to locate and tie-off the leaking artery that had been so painfully pumping blood into my muscle through the night.

Between gulps of nitrous oxide – I could hardly think of it as laughing gas under these circumstances – I knew the signs. I too had sweated involuntarily when faced with a difficult surgical task. The young houseman was beading-up nicely. Will I ever be able to find this bleeder? More probing: now next to the sensitive periosteum, the membrane covering the bone of my femur. Will it never end? Success at last! I don't know who was the more relieved. The offending vessel was ligated and I was hooked up for a blood transfusion. I had had enough, but my ordeal wasn't to end there.

A few minutes into my transfusion I began to experience unbearable itching in my groin and armpits. Before long I was pleading for the nurse to fetch a doctor. Even in my enfeebled state I knew that I was having a potentially dangerous anaphylactic reaction to the blood entering my body. I couldn't believe her response:

'I'm sorry, you'll have to wait. The doctors are having lunch at the moment.'

I was too ill to argue, but my condition spoke for me. I tore uncontrollably at my intensely wealing skin. Eventually I was disconnected from the 'bad' blood and properly treated for anaphylactic shock.

In the end my timing proved immaculate, and I recovered sufficient health to witness an uplifting event, the joy of which transcended the preceding unpleasant saga. Morwenna, our second daughter, was safely delivered in the maternity ward of the same hospital just a few days later.

Medical misadventure is a common occurrence, and the sort of experience I have outlined not uncommon. To my mind the only truly disquieting part was the response of the nurse to my blood transfusion reaction. The rest was a matter of bad luck. Sometimes unseen arteries can start bleeding after surgery; sometimes a pressure bandage is not enough to make them stop. Sometimes the consequence of a seemingly minor indiscretion may lead to death. I had seen it myself. I had caused it myself. Who am *I* to judge?

CHAPTER TWENTY-NINE

SOLD ON SOUTHLAND

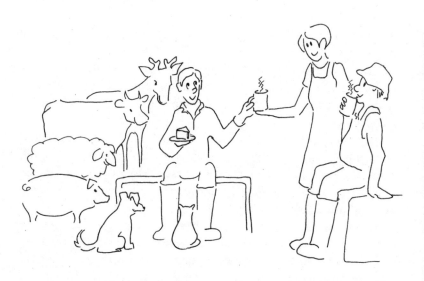

The farmer committee of the vet club for which I was working asked me to stay on once my period as a locum had ended, and I was duly appointed senior vet (of two). During six weeks of spring Viv and I had survived Southland's undoubtedly robust climate. It was, however, significantly milder than weather to be experienced even in the south of England, and so the climate wasn't an issue for us. Moreover, we had found myriad compensations and the decision to stay on was not difficult. Why? The hospitality of the locals is a good starting point. Almost invariably, whenever I finished a farm job, I was invited in for a cup of tea, often accompanied by home baking. The world is a busier place these days, but Southland hospitality is still a byword. The work was very varied and a day which could incorporate dairy or beef cattle, sheep, deer, cats, dogs and even the odd pig appealed to me. Any horse work seemed to involve children's ponies or farm hacks – still widely used on the larger farms for stock work. Most of the small-animal side involved working dogs. The toy repair stuff was minimal, an interesting side dish to other work rather than an overwhelming main course.

The working dogs are usually heading dogs, strong-eyed dogs of the familiar Border Collie type, or Huntaways – larger black and tan dogs which bark and push sheep ahead of them. Injuries are common, given the nature of their work. Broken legs, lacerations or torn ligaments are generally borne with stoicism by working dogs but Huntaways, in particular, have a wonderful temperament and it is generally a pleasure to work with them and their owners. They are far more biddable than many so-called pets and their owners are more down-to-earth and realistic in their expectations than the average city pet owner.

There was one drawback; I was now on a one-in-two duty roster. Nevertheless, the after-hours work was fairly minimal. A rrrring seldom disturbed our slumbers. I had previously found that farmers employing vets were respectful of after-hours time and tended to look after 'their' vets. It was part of the national ethos. Overseas visitors reported that New Zealand closed for the weekend. Not so good for visitors, but excellent for families. New Zealand has since joined the modern world and services are available at all hours. Veterinary practices in the towns compete with each other and hold routine evening, Saturday and Sunday clinics. Great for the spectators. Shame about the players.

In time the club employed three vets and, later still, after I joined in with a partner to lease the practice from the club, we expanded more. With an influx of dairy farmers in the early nineties the demand for veterinary services increased dramatically and, where there were two vets, there are now seven.

Over the years it has been my pleasure to work with many characters. The qualities which make a good large-animal vet: erudition, competitiveness, physical toughness, equability of temperament, combine in all of them in various proportions. But it is the capacity for humour that is most prized in the workplace.

Sooner or later as a vet, you will end up with egg on your face, or something a lot worse. Every one of the five senses will be periodically assailed, singly or in combination, as you will have gathered. Humour is the only balm, sometimes at your own expense, sometimes at someone else's. For starters I will highlight assaults to the first cranial nerve, which deals with olfaction, our sense of smell.

Kit was prepared to tolerate the idiosyncrasies of his uncontrolled dog, Steelo. Being a Labrador type, Steelo had eyes bigger than his stomach. He always accompanied Kit in his car. It was often a surprise to find out what he had found to eat while his master calved a cow or dealt with a lame horse, but find out we did as it usually fetched-up, in a partially digested state, on the carpet. It is not easy to remove the stench of a regurgitated rotten cow placenta that has had time to develop an intimate relationship with the soft furnishings of your car. Trading-in such a vehicle becomes problematical: especially now that the Privacy Act precludes doctors supplying lists of patients with severe olfactory lobe damage who could be potential buyers.

Another vet who was notorious for the untidy and noxious contents of his car was the butt of a rather unsubtle prank. Silage smells can be particularly demanding in the open air, let alone the enclosed confines of a car. To the average driver a wad of silage placed under his seat would be a noticeable addition to the interior milieu, especially on cold winter days, with the heater up and the windows closed. But Andy was not discomfited in the least. The olfactologist removed the evidence unremarked and undetected several days later after Andy had survived his trial by nose. No point in continuing, the silage was losing its potency. I dread to imagine what was tried next.

I have already alluded to competitiveness. By nature, vets tend to watch their patch fairly carefully. To vets with ego, it is unimaginable that any of their clients would stoop to use another vet. It is indeed upsetting for any vet to find out that they are not invariably the chosen one but, in a world of declining loyalties, it is the consumers' right to chop and change as they see fit. Vets must be constantly aware of this, because mistakes can arise if conflicting medication is given for the same patient by two different vets. Professional guidelines insist that the second vet involved contacts the preceding vet to establish the best course of action for the animal concerned. Vets who don't work in with their colleagues lay themselves open to a charge of 'supersession'. Unfortunately, some vets can't resist the opportunity to run down their opposition under such circumstances. "Of course, if I'd seen him in the first place... " Dr Shortfuse, the name given to one such individual by a Canterbury friend, was a pastmaster at this and not particularly popular with neighbouring vets.

The scene unfolds as Dr S arrives at my friend's practice for an appointment to sort out a dispute about supersession. He is getting decidedly puffy as he waits to see his colleague. He paces the waiting room, nostrils flaring. They were keeping him waiting deliberately. With time to kill he notices that the day book is prominently displayed. All part of the plan. He leans over the desk. Few vets could resist glancing to see what the opposition is doing. He catches a familiar name. Why are this crowd gelding colts for his favourite breeder? And further down, branding colts for another of his clients. More and more familiar names appear. Names of clients he thought he alone serviced. All part of the plan. That page of the day book was but an artifice, a fictional list doctored (not vetted) for the sole purpose of getting under Dr S's skin. It is not a good idea to go into a meeting in an irascible state and Dr Shortfuse had not acquired his nickname for nothing. He had his come-uppance that day.

Thus we reveal ourselves, not far removed from our schoolboy pasts.

But some are above all this, for they are not political animals. They are doers. A man in this category leaps on to these pages for a first appearance. I present my erstwhile partner, Daryl – sometime deer culler, deer farmer, sheep farmer, hunter, diver, whitebaiter and veterinarian. A man wedded to the outdoors. It was Daryl who was the first vet employed by the farmers' vet club and created a veterinary presence in an isolated rural area. He tackled tasks at which a more cautious Brit-type personality, such as me, would have baulked. In the early seventies he was single-handedly performing surgical embryo-transplant work on beef cattle, a technically and logistically demanding procedure, and achieving top results. He had the support of entrepreneurial farmers of integrity and a relatively litigation-free environment. These days such pioneering fieldwork would be stifled by legal considerations, the costs of indemnity insurance and a different class of assertive entrepreneur wanting quicker returns.

After a few years of farming and specialising in deer work Daryl was ready to become a full-time vet again. It was my good luck that I had his drive and positivity with me when we formed our partnership. Both of us refinanced to lease the practice from the club. The challenge of running our own business and shaping our own destinies was one we eagerly embraced. Though Daryl, of pragmatic farming stock, would no doubt put it in less flowery language.

'I mean, what is all this "embracing" and "destinies" stuff? It was a straightforward business deal.'

It was another step on life's journey as a practising vet.

CHAPTER THIRTY

REPRODUCTION REVISITED

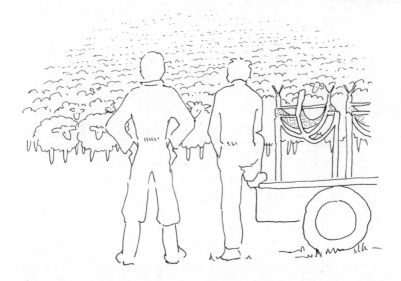

One of Daryl's most admirable traits is his willingness to tackle the largest jobs. His work output was remarkable. Pregnancy-testing cattle, blood-testing rams, develvetting deer: no one else could do the numbers as slickly as Daryl. Being naturally competitive, he liked to stay ahead of the rest of us in the pack. Then one day a truly gargantuan challenge fell in his lap.

Artificially inseminating cows is such a standard procedure that its importance tends to be overlooked. Semen from a top bull can be stored and transported in a frozen state around the world. The semen from a single ejaculate can be divided to fertilise dozens of cows. Most dairy and many beef cows undergo this annual ritual.

A technician suitably attired in shit-proof clothing: arm-length rubber gloves, plasticised jacket, over-trousers and gumboots – all readily available at your local menswear store – advances on the chosen cow. The left arm is inserted into the cow's rectum. Once there, the cervix is identified through the rectal wall and gently but firmly grasped. The right hand, holding a long pipette containing a straw of semen, now inserts the tip of the pipette into the cow's vagina and advances it towards the cervix. The pipette is manipulated through the cervical canal and the semen is deposited in the uterus ready to seek out and fertilise any eggs hanging about. What the cow thinks of all this is a matter of conjecture. I like the conjecture of one Henry Burgess:

I have just given birth to a heifer
of pride and milk I am full
But sad to relate – my pregnant state
was not brought about by a bull

How drab are the farmyards and meadows
Life seems empty and grey
For one bit of fun – on life's dreary run
Has by science been taken away

I have never been naughty – I swear it
In spite of the calf I have borne
Like farmer Brown's tractor – I'm 'virgo intacto'
I have not had a bull by the horn

It must not be thought that I'm jealous
There are things that a cow shouldn't say
But the 'land army tarts' who handle our parts
Get theirs – the 'old fashioned way'

Artificially inseminating sheep presents different problems. Most people are aware that sheep are somewhat smaller than their bovine cousins and there is currently a dearth of suitably trained gnomes to undertake the task. Although techniques have been developed to deposit semen in the cervix with a special pipette, conception rates are higher if it can be placed in the uterus itself, particularly if frozen semen is being used. It is just that little bit more debilitated by its long sleep in liquid nitrogen at −196°C.

For sheep, the only way to implant semen directly into the uterus involves using a laparoscope. A laparoscope is a long metal telescope linked to a fibre-optic light source which can be inserted into the abdominal cavity through a stab incision and used to locate the uterus. Meanwhile, via a second incision, a pipette is introduced and the semen injected through the wall of the uterus. It requires much practice and good hand/eye co-ordination to achieve this.

Laparoscopic AI is a surgical procedure requiring the ewe to be given a pain-killing sedative, strapped into a specially designed crate, and her belly to be shorn and disinfected as for any other surgery. With an efficient team of assistants and good facilities it is possible for a skilled operator to do about fifty ewes an hour. Daryl's challenge was to inseminate *sixteen thousand* ewes.

Farmers, disillusioned with poor lamb prices, were prepared to set aside a portion of their ewes for insemination with semen from Awassi rams. Awassis are a fat-tailed breed of sheep and the resulting half-bred lambs would fetch a premium price in Arab countries.

It was indeed fortunate that both Daryl and I had been trained up and had previously done some laparoscopic AI work, but I suspected that with my plodding twenty to thirty ewes an hour we would be struggling. I thought back to the difficulties I had had to begin with, when even ten or so an hour was an immense struggle, especially if the ewes were in good condition. The heavier a ewe is, the more difficult it is to find the uterus amongst billowing folds of fat-laden tissue inside her, and the less space there is to manipulate organs out of the way to obtain good access for the injection. Concentration at this level is draining and exhausting.

'How the hell are we going to do 16,000 ewes in less than a month at locations all over the lower half of the South Island?' I asked, not unreasonably.

'Yes, I was talking to the vets who have got the contract for the North Island. They reckon there's no way in the world that just two of us could do it. They offered to send a team of their vets down to do some of the farms, because they'll have finished their contract before us.'

That, of course, was all the challenge Daryl needed. He continued, 'I told them "no way", we have two vets experienced in laparoscopic AI and an excellent back-up team.'

The last statement turned out to be true and by the end of a month the former claim could justifiably be made. I wasn't to know this before we began, but despite my reservations I admired Daryl's 'can do' attitude. Besides which, the income was needed. The sheep industry and our business were facing a recession.

We cleared it with our other partners. They too would be under pressure holding the fort. Then we hit the trail. It was a month of hard work, but great enjoyment, as we set up in woolsheds around gloriously scenic parts of the country, and enjoyed the wonderful hospitality of the finest group of people you could wish to meet. Take a bow, New Zealand sheep farmers. In your sheds I have seen sweat and laughter, been plied with mouse-traps and the finest scones and, through the doors, refreshed my mind and spirit with the cool breezes drifting from snowy, sunlit peaks.

After each session Daryl and I would tally up. I feigned to take no interest. Daryl had always done a few more than I had. One session I felt I had had a particularly good run. Glenda, my assistant, counted my tally. 159. Not bad for two-and-a-half hours.

'How many, Daryl?' I asked confidently.

'A hundred and sixty-one', Daryl's assistant replied. That was as close as I ever got.

In the evenings, back in the country pubs, we relaxed over the pool table. Funny, but Daryl always seemed to win there too. Since he has semi-retired I shall now publicly acknowledge that Daryl is a winner, always has been. I couldn't have wished for a better partner. I didn't mind losing.

CHAPTER THIRTY-ONE

MOON METAL MADNESS

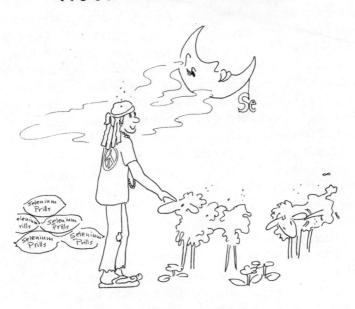

Without selenium, livestock farming in many parts of New Zealand would be impossible. Selenium is a trace mineral required by all mammals as an essential component of an enzyme. Without it, immune systems fail and muscles seize up. The heart is a muscle, so the consequences can be drastic. As with other trace elements there are endlessly variable symptoms depending on the depth of the deficiency and steepness of decline into the deficient state. Paradoxically it is possible to give too much and the end result of excess can be just as severe as deficiency. Selenium is a cumulative poison and in some parts of the world poisoning of livestock by plants that have the ability to concentrate selenium in their leaves is common.

At this stage I find it necessary to digress briefly into the realms of chemistry. Selenium is an element. It happens to be a metal.

Since it is not a carbon-containing compound, it is an *inorganic* chemical. Other essential inorganic chemicals include salt and water. Compounds that contain carbon chains are *organic* chemicals. Life on this planet is based on organic carbon-chain molecules. But there are many toxic organic chemicals ranging from naturally-produced poisons to artificially-synthesised pesticides. DDT is an organic chemical, but it is synthesised, not natural. Nicotine, caffeine and a host of other toxins naturally occur in plants and herbal remedies. Natural is not necessarily safe! Organic is not necessarily safe!

'Organic' farmers are bound by certain rules, depending on the body to which they subscribe. Some organisations permit them to resort to inorganic remedies, many of them toxic (copper, arsenic, selenium), but will not permit organic treatments or preventatives (such as synthetic pyrethroids, which are based on the naturally-occurring insecticide pyrethrum).

These days, before it can be registered for use, any synthesised drug has to be extensively trialled and data presented which closely establish efficacy, side-effects and persistence of residues. Thus a conventional farmer with lousy sheep may decide to use a synthetic pyrethroid pesticide to treat them for lice. The consumer is protected in the knowledge that the decay rates for these compounds are known and any meat and wool from treated animals will have minimal residues because there is a withholding period before treated animals can be sent for slaughter, policed by spot checks for residues. The organic farmer is limited to the natural product pyrethrum, derived from plants of the genus Chrysanthemum. The natural product will vary in concentration and efficacy depending from where it is sourced, and there will be no accompanying residue persistence data. It really is a punt in the dark.

Much of the organic debate is founded on absurd misapprehension. Above the foundations, the edifice is equally suspect. I would not wish to topple the general aim of those desiring so-called 'organic' produce if it minimises pesticide use (against external parasitic infestations) and conserves the use of antibiotics (against bacterial infections) and anthelminthics (against internal parasites). Ultimately, all those involved in arable or pastoral farming should be encouraged into sustainable practices. This does not preclude the use of pesticides (organic chemicals) in an informed manner with due cognisance of persistence and residues.

It has to be acknowledged that the rantings of some in the green lobby are frighteningly ignorant. Recently a New Zealand member of parliament for the Green party was, in a trick which revealed her ignorance, persuaded to campaign against the widespread use of dihydrogen monoxide in agriculture and the production of foodstuffs. This chemical, it was claimed, was being fed to livestock, despite being a component of precancerous cells. Even a novice chemist would recognise dihydrogen monoxide (H_2O) as water – essential to all life: a major component of *all* cells!

On the other hand, the use and marketing of synthetic chemical compounds has often been irresponsible and even corrupt in the hands of large multinational companies. The environmental damage caused by widespread use of persistent organochlorides such as DDT around the world in the fifties, sixties and seventies, the Thalidomide debacle, and misuse of hormones in meat production have justifiably resulted in increased awareness and tighter controls. There will always be a place for *informed* green politics.

You may have noticed that I have stopped bandaging dogs' paws and dabbling with cows' genitalia for a few paragraphs. There isn't much to laugh about with deltamethrin, no romance in benzimidazoles, little excitement in oxytetracyclines; but these molecules are at the core of being a vet. The dog with fleas, the horse with bots, the fawn with lungworm, and the cow with pneumonia, all require a chemical treatment. Any vets dealing with farm animals these days have to be fully aware, not only of the curative or preventative properties of the drugs they prescribe, but also of residues and withholding periods. The penalties for farmers caught flouting the regulations are very severe. The consumer is well protected these days, even if the produce doesn't bear an organic label.

Let us dispense with logic, efficacy and safety, and hark back to the good old days, when there where none of these nasty chemicals around. There were no antibiotics before the Second World War; all hospitals had septic wards. Some infections could be treated with, for instance, mercury compounds. Mercury, a heavy metal that made hatters mad. No anaesthetics till chloroform and ether came along – both dangerous till more effective replacements were synthesised. No effective anthelminthics: sheep were drenched with tobacco mixes and calves were injected with turps into their windpipes to cure lungworm. No pesticides for lice: people messed about

175

with butter and Stockholm tar 'salving' sheep until arsenical dips came along. They were very effective, but no one could describe arsenic as safe.

The moon metal. Selenium. Named after the Greek moon-goddess, Selene. Essential trace element. Toxic in excess. Nice name. If you're an organic farmer, tip it on. You may not be permitted to use vaccines to prevent deaths in your sheep or cattle, for reasons that defy logic, but selenium is not an issue. I would put in a plea for monitoring tissue levels to ensure a correct and safe rate, but that would offend beliefs that are anti-science. Put it in cow horns and bury it at the right phase of the moon. There's the romance. There's the mystery. But I warrant you'll rely on your trusty internal combustion engine to get you to your next organic producers' meeting, you'll promote your product on a website, and it will be wrapped in plastic on the supermarket shelves. The clock can only be turned back so far.

I firmly believe that if we really want to save this planet, feed the teeming millions *and* promote sustainability, we need more science, not less. For the individual farmer that means more investment in monitoring stock performance so that chemical inputs can be reduced to an effective minimum. Biotechnology is already delivering tools that we can use to reduce our reliance on toxic chemicals. For instance, genetic markers identifying sheep that are more naturally resistant to diseases will, by a simple blood test, enable a farmer to know which rams to use over his ewes. If he can breed sheep that are more resistant to worms, he will use less drench. The farm-animal vet has an increasingly important role at the interface between the farmer and new technologies, which will truly help us to 'green' the livestock industries.

CHAPTER THIRTY-TWO

REDWATER REVERIES

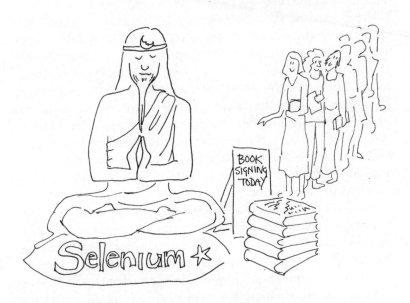

A fair part of the summer months in our practice is occupied by pregnancy-testing dairy cows. This seemingly unglamorous task involves inserting a gloved and lubricated arm into the cow's rectum and palpating her uterus. Thousands of cows are tested over the course of a few months, and although the job has been made easier for large herds by the use of electronic scanners, we are essentially what one of my colleagues refers to as 'bum-hole technicians'. It is a seemingly thankless task, but it helps the bank balance. Manual pregnancy testing is one of those hard-won skills. It takes a lot of practice for a vet to acquire the ability to assess the stage of pregnancy, detect uterine infections and manipulate the ovaries to check for abnormalities that could be causing infertility. It is also physically demanding. The operator is doing a variation of one-armed push-ups many times over, often while balancing on a wobbly plank placed in the pit of the milking shed. The cow's anal sphincter resents the intrusion and clamps down painfully on burning muscles. The bigger and more muscular the arm, the more effort required. Until relatively recently, the odd 'colour therapist' was around – diagnosing pregnancy in cattle by swinging a gold ring tied to a horse hair over the cow's back; and of course, he was right some of the time!

Depending on the set-up, an experienced vet can pregnancy test around a hundred cows an hour. As herd sizes grew, Daryl and I were processing up to six- or 700 cows at a time. Two- or 300 is a pleasant physical challenge, six- or 700, a long and painful ordeal. As the practice expanded we had more vets available and if there were more than two-hundred to do we could send out two vets. With electronic scanners, the boundaries have been pushed further and a thousand cows can be scanned in the four hours it takes to milk them. It is still very hard work: a game that advancing age has graciously enabled me to pass on to the fitter and more beautiful members of our practice.

If you are right-handed it is supposedly easier to learn to palpate with the left. Since the fingers of my left hand had been severed in that skill-saw accident, I had had to relearn with my right but, as the sensory innervation returned, I eventually found I could use either hand. I enjoyed building on this basic defining skill, the very essence of being a respected large-animal vet.

Share with me the day I was happily pregnancy testing the last of fifty heifers for Ego Centric. I was indulging my honed skills and the farmer had a good result.

'Gosh, you should be really pleased Ego. Every one in calf and only one a bit late. You've beaten the law of averages.'

'Yeah, right. But I'd like to talk to you about that calf problem before you go.'

By this stage I had cleaned up my gear and was seeking some sanctuary to escape and empty my bladder. Yes, even vets have to urinate at times and although farm animals, and some farmers, let fly anywhere within the farm boundaries, an inner modesty inclines me to be more inhibited.

Daryl was fond of recounting the time he descended a long driveway down a river terrace. As he started his drive down he noticed the farmer hunched up against a fence, down by the woolshed, in that familiar posture. He was still there as Daryl drew up beside him. Not suspecting the farmer might have prostate trouble Daryl (tactfully?) remarked, 'That was a bloody long piss!' The rejoinder, 'Well I've got a bloody long cock!' is one of those morning tea-time classics.

The incident at Ego Centric's was marginally less humorous for me.

'Look Ego, excuse me a second while I have a leak.' I ducked behind a wall. Noting my aim I was at first surprised, then alarmed to see scarlet splashes on the wall. I was peeing blood. This was more than the after-effects of a beetroot binge. Although the emissions of my bladder are not a topic I would regularly share in conversation, in this instance I felt impelled to express my alarm – perhaps to self-indulgently receive just a morsel of human sympathy in return.

'By crikey, Ego, I've just pissed a whole heap of blood.'

Haematuria wasn't on Ego Centric's agenda at all.

'Yeah, but you look OK. What about these calves? I've got to be in town in half an hour.'

And so I did the professional thing and saved my worries till I was in the car driving home.

~

Over the next few years I was destined to increase my acquaintance with my urinary system and, in particular, my urethra. This tiny pipe connection between the bladder and the outside world plays a part in human affairs wholly incommensurate with its size. It is the urethra, pulsing at a frequency of zero point eight of a second, which is responsible for the rapture of orgasm. The human pizzle is a highly sensitive and delicate organ. If your doctor, in the course of his investigations, thrusts a cottonwool swab down your urethra, he will elicit a response. I can vouch for it.

The swab was negative. I had no earthly reason to suspect I had VD, but doctors are dealing with all sorts of people these days and I couldn't begrudge mine the fun of eliminating this important differential diagnosis. X-rays and a CT scan followed, revealing the true culprit. A tumour growing in my bladder. This was the big C that everyone dreads. A transitional cell carcinoma. The last word snarls from the page for anyone with even a passing familiarity with pathology. This was a malignant cancer. It had to be removed forthwith. The prognosis – an eighty per cent chance of survival after five years. Rather worse than I would have anticipated in the normal course of events. Think of a number between one and five. Rather worse than Russian roulette. You mustn't get negative, John.

What had I done to deserve this? I asked not for reasons of self-pity, but out of pure interest. This was a disease pre-eminently of smokers. I didn't smoke. It afflicts those in the printing industries, those working with dyes and rubber tyres and it could manifest many years after exposure to the initiating toxins. Blame it on a childhood cycling the streets of Liverpool – to and from school, to and from university – quaffing the leaden exhaust fumes from myriad diesel trucks and buses. Unlikely. There would be no bladders left in Merseyside if this theory was a starter. No one had an *inkling*, but in this strange little word lies a clue. We must go back to Junior school to understand my theorem.

~

'All right children: pen, pencil, ruler, rubber, blotting paper.' On Mrs Beattie's command the whole class dutifully held up these items. Woe betide anyone who couldn't display them. Who would want to stay back during morning break to write lines? Try writing 'I must remember to bring my blotting paper' fifty times in copper-plate, using a scratchy steel dip-in nib on inferior-grade paper, *and no splotches*. Mrs Beattie meant what she said and her class was always well-behaved. For me, in hindsight, the unimaginative teaching methods were somewhat compensated by the romance of belonging to that last generation of schoolchildren to use the ancient paraphernalia of nibs and inkwells, but I was not aware of these sensitivities at the time.

There were other traditions to uphold. Every master wore a gown. Black and crow-like they stalked the school in these medi-aeval crimped smocks, mysterious assemblages of false sleeves and dangling be-knotted and be-buttoned ties: wafting down the corridors, congregating in the cloisters, lurking in the library, patrolling the playing-fields or caning in the classrooms – alliteratively alert to every minor schoolboy indiscretion.

Stevo, our maths teacher, was a gruff but kind-hearted man, with a slow fuse of anger that we boys could light on occasions. After the restrictions of double English with Mrs B, the temptations to create a diversion were impelling and Stevo often suffered the consequences of our restless little spirits.

As he slowly paced down the aisles between our desks, appraising our progress on the problem he had set us, he had no cause to delay long over my blank page. The dapper and intelligent Ellis, in front of me, was more worthy of his help. Stevo's black, scholastic drapery glided across my desk as he bent to his task. I swear I only had to move that button an inch to hook it into a triangular break on the edge of my bakelite inkwell. Inevitably, as Stevo moved on, the full inkwell slid up Ellis' back and decanted over his shoulder – despite my self-serving warning cries. A blue-black birthmark spread over Ellis' pristine grey shirt.

Oh calamity! Indeed, I think these were the very words Stevo uttered as he spun round, arcing the ink onto yet another desk. There was plenty of work for boys rushing to assist with blotting paper. Despite their best efforts I suspect Mrs Ellis was not best pleased at the end of the day; however, right now, Stevo was starting to lose his grip. An early version of paint-ball, involving rulers and ink-soaked pellets of blotting paper, was evolving behind his back every time he addressed the blackboard. It was when one hit him on the neck that he finally flipped. Bellowing and red-faced, caught between jumping up and down with rage and running to deal with the miscreants, he bounced, kangaroo-style, to the back of the class. There, in a frenzy of flailing bat wings and a flurry of papers, two boys were belted savagely about their heads. Just as suddenly the storm passed. A saddened, careworn man whispered apologies for his human failings and departed the room. We never even found out how many oranges the Chinaman could fit in the box, although I was more interested in the accompanying illustration in the textbook and wondered why his pigtail didn't get caught in the spokes of his bicycle.

We became no less cruel as we became seniors, though we progressed from steel nibs and inkwells to fountain pens. The fun and mess of ink diminished, and as we matured we became more materialistic. With a luminous wristwatch and an elegant Parker pen, the average schoolboy was as happy as today's teenager with a cellphone and an Xbox.

I treasured my blue Parker pen with its gold nib and used it right through my university years. I polished the nib with blotting paper till it gleamed and, by a strange compulsion, I was occasionally drawn to sip the ink – a repellent, salty tang – challenging and forbidden. Of course, it would never happen these days. Every bottle will come with a health notice warning of the dangers of drinking or gargling with ink, and to use a double-thickness glove technique before writing with the stuff. You can't even buy a car without a bible-thick manual warning you not to chew on the doors in case you damage your dentures, and any other possibly damaging permutation of bizarre behaviour which could lead your lawyers to claim against the manufacturer. Ink ingestion as a youth could have been a contributory cause to my bladder cancer. How silly of me.

~

Thank goodness for modern medical science. In the hands of an expert that first tumour was removed via a cystoscope not very different from the laparoscope I had inflicted on those ewes. The cystoscope is inserted up the dilated urethra and the whole proce-dure performed within the bladder. As I awoke from my anaesthetic it was the insult to my urethra of which I was first aware. What's more, an impossibly large plastic tube was keeping it stretched to pass the inevitable blood clots ensuing from the operation site. A few days hovering between extreme discomfort and pain and then this wretched catheter could be removed. That was when I knew the true meaning of pain, or I thought I did.

Life went on. Every three months new tumours were detected in my bladder and the same procedure followed. Occasionally post-operative blood clots created total blockages and I underwent emergency ambulance dashes to the hospital. Most importantly I witnessed others in far worse predicaments than I was. A stay in hospital generally removes any vestiges of self-pity. Then one day, with the threat of radiotherapy imminent, my check-up was clear. My urethra had survived, slightly distended, but still very serviceable.

It wasn't to be the end of our battle with cancer.

~

Yes, it was *our* battle. I drew strength from the courageous support of a loving wife. It involved both of us and we had two dependent teenage children. 'Soul-searching' is a much-used cliché, but it was vigorously applied as we adjusted to the changing prognoses. Good health becomes a precious commodity when it can no longer be relied upon. We learned to celebrate our blessings daily: the strength of our relationship, the pride we had in our two healthy daughters, the beauty of our surroundings, and our health. We aimed for, and I believe we achieved, a state of serenity which has not left us, though it has been sorely tested.

Of interest in all this is the psychology of cause and effect. If you take positive action – pray for deliverance, or start on a course of blue-green algae – and your condition resolves, is the cure a result of your action, or would it have happened anyway? I have a fair idea that my reprieve can be attributed to modern medicine. But *How I Beat Cancer by Heeding Medical Advice* will never be a bestseller.

To all those who are adamant that they have won their battles with cancer by fighting it in their minds, by adopting a vegan diet, by seeking endless second opinions and referrals, by adopting new religious beliefs – well good luck to you, but don't go foisting your illogical baggage on the rest of us. It disturbs my state of serenity.

Perhaps because of such obdurate attitudes, it seems that I was selected for a second bout with C. This time a small tumour appeared unheralded at the back of my mouth one New Year's Day – an auspicious discovery. Another malignancy: this time a squamous cell carcinoma. Once again I was at the mercy of the surgeons. Prognosis with prompt removal: once again, eighty per cent after five years. Take two of those and the odds are shortening; my luck may run out one of these days. Time to review lifestyles. Time to re-invent myself. Appearing in a local newspaper near you...

Jon Hix [pictured in thoughtful and sincere pose with flowing Manchu-style beard and orange toga] *has returned from many years of study under Lunarian monks in Outer Magnolia. Jon's* move was inspired after miraculous recoveries from two types of malignant cancer. He initially attributed this to his ability to attain a state of serenity. However, a dyslexic New Zealand 'colour therapist' convinced him that the word serene transposed with selene for Asiatic speakers of English. This amazing co-incidence and his previous professional life as a veterinarian working with selenium-deficient animals convinced him to travel to Magnolia at the behest of the aforesaid dyslexic. Furthermore Jon knew that sheep deficient in selenium, 'the Moon metal', were prone to adenocarcinomata – malignant cancers of the small bowel. Obviously there was some link between the moon and a cure for cancer.

Jon has now returned to set up a clinic to give Western cancer sufferers the chance to undergo the ancient healing rituals of 'Lunatic Therapy', the object of which is to attain a state of 'lunacy'. Adepts can advance into 'sheer lunacy', at which stage their cancers will appear unimportant to them and even their loved-ones will cease to care.

Jon's new book How I Beat Cancer by Joining the Lunatic Fringe is currently a bestseller.

CHAPTER THIRTY-THREE

MONEY FOR NOTHING AND THE KICKS FOR FREE

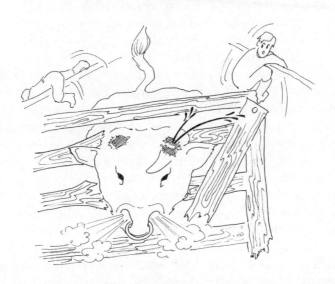

In a working life dealing with large animals it is inevitable that at some stage a close escape is going to turn into an accident. Many accidents happen because of inadequate facilities, but the temptation is to complete the job rather than decline it and get back in your car. For younger vets there is even more pressure. 'I don't know what you're complaining about. Bud has been doing it behind that gate for years.' On arrival back at the clinic you take issue with Bud. 'I agree with you, John. I've been telling him to install a decent head-bail for years.'

A head-bail is a device, usually of strong metal pipe construction, that clamps a cow or bull by the neck. For any procedure a vet or farmer has to do involving the head or front end of a bull it is almost indispensable. It is possible to make do with a rope halter round the head, but that in turn has to be secured to an immovable object, and that was where my system was about to fail.

The object of my attentions was a frisky Jersey bull. Even 'Slow' Lerner had decided that it was time to put a ring in his nose and dehorn him. But 'Frisky', who had until now enjoyed free dominion, was extremely displeased with the constraint of the rope halter that we had somehow managed to drop over his head. From one side of a gate we slowly played him in, like a prize tuna, till he was adjacent to the gate of a milking bail, and then hitched him up to it as tightly as we could. Like most facilities on Slow's farm it was apparent that this gate was approaching senescence. But it was to suffer no slow descent into oblivion.

With great difficulty I injected the local anaesthetic nerve blocks to desensitise the horns before I cut them off with a saw. Frisky rattled his head against the gate trying to pin my hand as I reached through the bars. There were angry prolonged bellows and he was pawing the ground. A fired-up bull at close range is an impressive sight. His struggles had already gained him about six inches of laxity as the rope stretched, and this gave him more leeway to batter the tottering gate. Somehow I managed to remove one horn, but the nerve block can't have taken properly on the other side. I was over half-way through when Frisky had had enough and decided to remove the rest himself by butting his head clean through the frail timbers. As he lunged and raised his head, the gate was lifted off its pins and we were faced with an unrestrained, rampant bull wearing a gate necklace. Slow had a three-foot start on Frisky. Mine was considerably less.

Behind us was a narrow concrete passageway through which the milked cows, on less pressing occasions, ambled contentedly to pasture. The concrete was slippery with moss and slime. The wall, seven feet of it, was the back wall for the shed and continued at the same height past the roofed area. It was only when we revisited the scene that I made these observations. Both of us had cleared that wall in a trice – testimony to the incredible reserves we can all draw on when that adrenalin surges in our blood – as Frisky clattered through beneath our feet. Slow was not so named for any physical incapacity.

Out in the paddock a maddened bull had finally cast off his wooden yoke and, in the surprising manner of such animals, had instantly settled once he was free. He was contentedly chewing the grass. With some trepidation I retrieved my strained halter, but Frisky wasn't really interested. Most dangerous animals are not malevolent. They don't hold personal grudges. They are just reacting to circumstances. If you happen to be in the way, well, look out!

~

Real accidents come out of the blue. I drove the long, straight Canterbury road to my next visit, to pregnancy-test a mare. There she was in the yard, already caught, and with Maggie holding a lead rope attached to her head collar. All ready to go then. This shouldn't take too long. Not as if I was going to have to frig around for half an hour trying to catch her first, as is so often the case on these hobby farms. A Welsh mountain pony hovered in the background. Maggie was devoted to her equine friends.

'Do you really need to hobble her? I don't want her hurt,' I was asked, as I slid the rope round her neck, tied the bowline and then looped the sidelines through hobbles on her rear fetlocks to stop her kicking me. It was the minimum I was prepared to do. All vets are brought up with stories of horrific injuries from kicks. Standing directly behind a mare with your arm in her rectum, an intrusion that many mares naturally resent, is putting yourself in a vulnerable position.

'That's one area where I won't take short cuts, Maggie,' I said firmly. The discomfort of the sidelines to her mare were more important to her than my safety. Time and again vets have to override this protective instinct in the pet-owning public.

'I think that if you had my job to do, you'd be the same. You might get away with it once, but eventually you'd be caught out.'

At this stage I was startled to see the mare's perineum contracting. In equine parlance she was 'winking', meaning she was probably on heat. A bit unusual. Mares on heat aren't usually pregnant. Maggie wouldn't have called me out if she had displayed such signs of heat earlier. I was all set up to examine her, so I may as well do a rectal examination while I was there. Sidelines secure... OK, here we go. The next minute I was delivered a fearful blow to my thigh and lay in breathless spasm on the ground. It wasn't the mare; it was that blasted Welsh mountain pony. It was a stallion. The mare *was* on heat. I was the competition, though I hadn't realised it. I hadn't even seen the little blighter sneak up on me. She was winking at him, not me!

Maggie helped me up. The pain eased. Nothing broken. In numbed discomfort I slowly unlooped the sidelines. Maggie had removed the little sod responsible for my injury. As with Frisky, he was not innately vicious. I had merely been competition in the wrong place at the wrong time.

I must have looked pale because Maggie, by now profusely apologetic, insisted I had a cup of tea. She really shouldn't have had that stallion wandering around loose in the yard and she knew it. Fortified by that sweet elixir I limped to my car. Fortunately the long, straight road home did not necessitate me to change gears too often, because my left leg was rapidly seizing up.

At last I reached the sanctuary of our driveway and that was where Viv found me ten minutes later.

'I thought I heard the car come in,' she said. Did I detect a slight tone of impatience? Yes!

'What on earth are you still sitting there for?' she continued.

'It's not my habit to sit in cars,' I rejoined. 'You know I only regard them as a means of conveyance. The fact is I can't move. Once again I've been nailed by one of those creatures so dear to your heart.'

This was an oblique reference to her misspent youth with ponies, one of which had trodden on my toe shortly before our wedding. (That bruise had become infected and the abscess under my large toe nail had played a significant part in our honeymoon – at one stage of which I had been rendered delirious with pain rather than the pleasure I had so eagerly anticipated.)

Somehow Viv managed to coax and manipulate me from the relatively pain-free refuge of my car seat and into the house. A massive haematoma in my quadriceps was surgically removed a few days later and after a week or so on crutches I was once again on the road.

I can still feel the calcified remains of that bruise, the largest they had seen at the hospital, or so they said. A couple of inches higher and the hoof would have connected with the bones of my hip and not the fleshy padding of my thigh. A shattered hip would have been far more serious. I had been lucky.

Frisky was an accident waiting to happen and these days neither I, nor any of our staff, would be expected to perform their job with unsafe facilities. My incident with Maggie's horse was the sort of accident that most vets occasionally experience. Despite being careful, most equine vets have been kicked, and every small-animal practitioner has been bitten or scratched at some stage. There is the occasional dog which attacks without warning, but usually the owner alerts you to that fact before you deal with his (it is, as a rule, a male thing) 'pet'. Even Barry Hardcastle may have been savaged by the odd guinea pig during his fictitious career. But perhaps the worst prospect is putting yourself in a position where you know there is a reasonable chance of getting a hiding. Most deer vets have had one.

Those vets who dealt with deer in the days when deer farming was a new venture will appreciate my sentiments. Farmers had yet to establish the optimal layout for deer yards. Some arrangements were diabolical: unroofed pens with high walls. Try concentrating on clipping a stag with a pair of noisy clippers while a couple of frantic 200-kilo companions repeatedly attempt to jump for freedom, not caring where and on whom they land when they bounce back into the pen.

Some farmers who had joined the cervine gold rush had no empathy with their animals and were unable to adjust to the different level of stockmanship required when working with deer. The worst of them were frightened of their animals.

The comment 'It's OK, John, I'll close the door', meant from the outside, leaving you alone with a heaving mass of hinds, a clipper and a tuberculin syringe.

Clippers are noisy, and already nervous animals can behave in unpredictable ways. Subordinate types crouch on the floor and there you have to follow, trailing the clipper cord behind you. This presents an opportunity for the aggressive dominant ones to have a go at you. None of this is a problem if you are supported by capable staff who look out for you as you concentrate on the job in hand, but there were some farms where we all dreaded going.

For the recipient of an attack by a stroppy deer the reality sinks in a few seconds later, so sudden is the assault. Your helmet and shoulders are peppered by a maelstrom of heavy blows and there she is; wild-eyed, trembling and hair on end, waiting to have another go.

Warily you keep other deer between you and her while your team, with luck, can draft her out of the pen. In a very crude way you have been reminded of human frailty. No matter how macho we are, our strength and reaction times are feeble compared to those of these wild animals honed by millennia of evolutionary adaptation. Our brain power, aided by medical advances, is surely taking humanity in the opposite direction on the evolutionary highway.

Too much adrenalin is wearying and a day spent assessing potential antagonists in pens full of angry deer is no picnic. Deer farmers now have better facilities, many with hydraulic crushes for large and fractious animals. 'Killer' deer are no longer valuable and are culled before they can become too much of a menace. More to the point, it has become a specialist business attracting those who know what they're doing. Hobbyists with a few deer and make-do pens manufactured from scraps of netting placed round a mud patch, with an off-cut carpet as a roof, have thankfully disappeared.

~

And so, if you are a large-animal vet the kicks *are* free, but what about the money? Here the analogy with the popular song fails. An employed veterinarian should enjoy a comfortable income for all his or her hard work and, if they become a partner or invest in their business, perhaps better (perhaps worse). Unfortunately there is always room for exploitation in a profession which many join for love. It would be a sad day were we to sink to the mores prevailing during the Great Depression, when 'gentlemen', keen to gain experience, would pay to work as a vet. A sad day for all of us.

My farming clients would no doubt disagree and, as second thoughts and from my position as partner in a veterinary business, I can feel myself warming to the idea.

CHAPTER THIRTY-FOUR

VALOUR AND DISCRETION

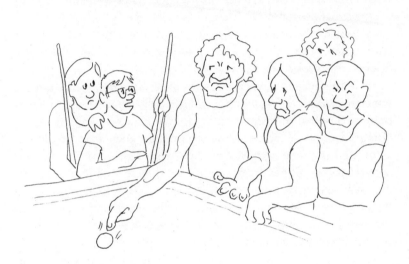

The crowd disgorges from the confines of the Kop and fans out across the streets: army ants on the move. Substitute the leaf litter of a forest floor for the stained tarmac of a Liverpool street, a beetle carcase dismembered and shouldered aside for that terrified couple hunched in their car as the army seethes round them – its soldiers reckless and untouchable in the frenzied knowledge of their united power. Above them bollards of mounted police represent law and order – a mere gesture – for where the press is thickest they are as powerless and immovable as tree trunks in that alien jungle.

Though the terrified couple do not know it they are in luck, for this is a good-natured swarm. Liverpool has had a home win and the army is in a playful mood. It contents itself with merely banging on the roof, and only for a brief moment is there a more sinister threat as a cadre positions itself fore and aft and gives the unsettled occupants a decent rocking. A few millimetres of glass separate them from these jeering louts. They adopt appeasing grimaces. It is a hopeless ploy, and they know they have no control over their destiny. Just as suddenly their tormentors lose interest and move on. Soon the car's occupants are able to furtively creep around the straggling remnants, rueing the timing that induced them to forage round the back streets of the stadium on this particular afternoon. With relief their motor accelerates them to freedom. The dented carapace can be repaired. It could have been so much worse.

As part of the army I had been caught up in the action. I had felt the dangerous euphoria of our united power. I had felt for the brief terror of our casually discarded prey.

Since this teenage experience I have registered extreme unease about any form of mass hysteria and its ability to suspend individual thought. Look at the frenzied participants in archived film from the Nuremburg rally; look at the unreasoned violence and chanting at massed political protests, or the divine rapture of evangelical congregations. These are all people who have sold their souls to a higher authority, invariably a human one, often claiming to be the mouthpiece of some supernatural god. Tell them to believe and they will. Command them to genocide and they will. Tell them to top themselves and they will. Remember Jonestown?

What would I have done if the crowd had turned ugly? What *could* I have done? It gave me immense respect for the courage of Bishop Desmond Tutu when he stepped in to rescue a victim from 'necklacing' by a lynch mob.

Of course Tom Brown would have done the same. Against all odds fictional heroes have stepped in and done their bit repeatedly and, usually unbelievably, survived. It makes the genuine real-life heroes, the Ernest Shackletons, Nancy Wakes and Charles Uphams, all the more admirable.

Not being a fictional character, and priding myself on a modicum of common-sense, I have never been the sort to march into a pub and pick a fight with the largest and ugliest at the bar, but I did wonder about Brian as we waited to meet a sales rep in an Ashburton pub. Ashburton is, to all outward appearances, a civilised little town. There are no docklands or bombed-out slums in Ashburton. To survive unharmed through a Liverpool childhood it was advantageous to avoid certain areas at certain times, to avoid looking at certain people in certain, undefined, ways. In general Liverpudlians are warm, friendly and humorous people, but the infamous 'Liverpool kiss' is no manifestation of affection.

Our rep wasn't showing up. (He had waited for us in vain in the Seaforth Lounge. 'I would never have gone to *that* bar.') Without trepidation we gravitated to the back of the room to have a quiet game of pool. A Maori shearing gang was occupying the table. Tough men and women lined the walls. They worked hard all day and they played hard each night. After several games the table was idle. Brian and I waited politely to see if anyone else wanted to play. No? We seized our opportunity, stepped up and put our money in the slot. We set up the balls and started to play. After several years in New Zealand I had dropped my guard. Premonitions to which my Liverpool upbringing would normally have alerted me no longer blipped my radar screen.

A lean, muscular man of monolithic proportions strode casually to our table and rolled the cue ball away from the shot I had lined up. It was *almost* accidental. But then he started to mess with the other balls. I abandoned my naivety. This was deliberate! Brian was the first to speak. As an aside, he stage-whispered to me, 'I never back down in situations like this'– just when I was considering that discretion would be the better part of valour. Well if he wasn't backing down, how could I?

I surveyed the opposition. We were outnumbered at least five to one by men obviously attuned to such situations. Intensely they focused on our little drama. Any conversation between them had ceased. Hands clenched on glasses and jugs. They were going to play this one out, and the Queensberry rules would have no part in it. They were quite obviously about to make mincemeat of us. Neither of us would be a match for men honed by a demanding physical job, men who sheared two- or 300 sheep a day – day in, day out. We might palpate a few rams, play the odd game of squash and do a spot of tramping. If it came to a stoush, we weren't in their league.

Monolith started to swear. Explosive 'f' and 'c' words filled the air. The rest of the room became expectantly quiet, a sea of white faces blobbing out of focus in my field of vision. Intently I concentrated on the epicentre of this aggressive tirade. Brian responded to the barrage of invective with a bald statement. 'You've got a rather limited vocabulary.'

It seemed rather a tactless thing to say. Internally I applauded the wry humour, but its subtlety was lost on Monolith who seemed to be in a world of his own. A rictus of wild indifference masked any shred of humanity. Eye contact was of the glazed variety. Nothing we said was going to register. He beckoned to his deputy, a smaller, shifty character. Belligerently he carried an empty jug towards us, poising it over the table. The implication was obvious. Adrenalin, the hormone of 'flight or fight', is a strange thing. We couldn't back down now. Flight was out. I prepared myself for the worst.

Our plight had not gone unobserved. In the nick of time three policemen walked into the pub. They made straight for the pool table.

'Everything OK here, guys?'

Monolith abandoned his zombie persona and a warm smile suffused his face. I have never seen such a rapid transformation. The police tried another tack and spoke directly to Monolith.

'We have reason to believe you're about to cause trouble again.'

'No, we're going to have a drink with these boys, officer.' He held his hand out to shake Brian's and then mine. The tension in the rest of the gang relaxed.

'What you having, boys?' Before we knew it jugs of beer were set in front of us and the police melted away. They had done a great job, courtesy of an observant publican.

Brian and I were next faced with a gargantuan and very amicable drinking session. The first drink was welcome, but more kept coming. How could we refuse? We didn't want to cause offence, yet Brian was determined to maintain the psychological upper-hand. The debate, such as it was, consensually visited such topics as the futility of violence, self-improvement through education, saving to benefit the future of your dependents. It was a bravura performance. For an hour or two we were all the best of mates. I wish I could remember more... We both returned home drunk that night. It could have been so much worse.

And yet, reflecting on this display of courage reminds me that, on another occasion, Brian was quite unable to face a rocky mountain ridge. Vertigo, fear of flying, arachnophobia: probe deep enough and every one of us has a weak point somewhere. I have had great personal difficulty confronting my own deep fears of happy-clappy congregations and country and western music. But I need to probe deeper than that.

~

My first day at boarding school was a shock. After a brief farewell to my parents at the front door, I was ushered by Mr Pratt into the front room of the Victorian residence – the Junior boarding school. Mr Pratt had been charming to my parents, but seemed decidedly distant once the front door was closed. Never mind, he was a busy man. It was old Pratt who supervised our ritual daily cold baths. It was old Pratt who caned each and every one of us when a boy was hospitalised with concussion after the traditional end-of-year pillow fight. He was a diligent man, determined to instil some good old-fashioned values into us and harden us up.

A group of boys were enjoying a roughhouse over and around the tatty furniture. They scarcely paused at my entrance, and resumed their play. In one corner another boy sat rather disconsolately. Perhaps he too had just been dropped off by his parents. I was keen to face the challenge of my new life, but even though we were only twelve- or thirteen-year-olds, I had enough understanding to empathise with the misery of a fellow human being. It wasn't till I started to approach him that any notice was taken of me.

'Don't talk to Evans.'

A solid boy, 'Hippo', was making a firm recommendation.

'Why not?' I asked.

'He's a coward.' The story was related to me while Evans shifted miserably in his corner.

The previous year Evans, for some reason, had called Wickham a 'bastard'. Wickham, as I was later to find out, fully justified that description. He was, for his age, a squat and powerfully built boy. He had had private boxing tuition in Jamaica, his home country. It would be easy to gauge that Evans, a skinny and incoordinated child, would be no match for Wickham. Wickham seized his opportunity for immortality. Choosing to interpret the term 'bastard' as impugning his mother's honour, he took the complaint to Mr Pratt. As a man of the old school, Mr Pratt was, or feigned to be, shocked. In a move that guaranteed him respect from the boys he acceded to Wickham's request and permitted a boxing match. He produced the gloves to make sure that everything was fair. This was the manly way to settle disputes.

Wickham smugly listened as Hippo recounted Evans' nemesis to me.

For the first round of that fight Wickham had toyed with Evans.

'You should have seen Evans at the end of the first round,' remembered Hippo with glee, 'his nose was pulped and there was blood all over his face.'

They cleaned him up. Evans was quite an obstinate boy. He had been given the opportunity to apologise and not realised the significance of not taking it. He had never been popular, or tried to seek popularity. His parents were missionaries in China, if they had known of their son's plight perhaps they would have thought it was excellent training for their line of business. It would be nice to think that they would have been horrified. Not so Mr Pratt.

He let the fight continue. After a further pummelling Evans made a mistake that would live with him for the rest of his school days; and, if *I* can remember it now, for the rest of his life. *He ran away from Wickham.* As long as any of these boys knew him, he would be labelled a coward. He was never going to redeem himself on the playing-field. He was at the bottom of the C form. His parents were on the other side of the world. He was a hopeless case, but by merely surviving in that poisonous atmosphere for a few years he showed more courage than most of his tormentors.

In divulging this tale of woe, Hippo seemed to be including me into his group. He was now going to show me the 'fifty-four card trick'. He grabbed a pack from the shelf. All eyes were on me.

'Go on. What is it then?' I asked eagerly. Hippo heaved the cards in the air.

'Now pick them up.'

I ignored him. I was by nature a tidy boy. I had always cleared up my toys after play. I glanced round the shabby room. Discarded magazines littered the floor. I suspected that a few greasy cards wouldn't make much difference. Anyway a bell sounded. Tea time! Without further ado Hippo and the other boys were squeezing through the door. He was a greedy bastard, although I never had the guts to say it to his face. He was bigger than me. I wasn't stupid. His demise would come later when he became stuck in a tarn at a Scout camp in the Wicklow mountains. The hatred of the past-bullied who united to lob stones and witness his disintegration under fire was a surprise to him. All they that take the sword shall perish with the sword. He was the better for realising it.

I suspect Wickham became a successful estate agent (after his holiday job as an assistant in a psychiatric institution where he avowedly was able to indulge his whims with mentally defective women) and Hippo a car salesman. As to Evans, I dread to think. After a few years of being unremittingly reviled he disappeared.

In a very short space of time I had learned that cowardice is an unpardonable indiscretion and it is perfectly acceptable, indeed endorsed by the authorities, to bully a coward in the most cowardly ways imaginable. We all need a scapegoat, someone lower on the pecking order whom we can legitimately despise.

I left the Junior boarding school a year later a wiser and more cynical boy. I was looking forward to Senior school and becoming one of the hardened elite in School House. I was about to step out of the frying pan and into the fire. Pernicious memories come flooding back.

~

Makliski, we failed you. Although you bunked for a year next to me, that is the only name by which I knew you. Oh yes! Your parents were recently separated and a few years later you were expelled. You were harmless, but you were different. When the older boys raided our dorm for a victim, it was you they chose. We individually cowered in relief that it was not one of us they carried to their dorm. And so it was you they tossed mercilessly in a blanket, indeed so hard that there were some awkward explanations to explain the exposed laths where your tensely terrified body had cracked the plaster off that high ceiling. Boys will be boys!

Repeatedly, you will note, I call on you, Tom Brown, a hero that my late-developing body never allowed me to emulate. Even at thirteen you would have shown them your mettle. Your prowess at the game your school gave name to was no joy to me. I never rejoiced in thrusting my head and shoulders between the foetid buttocks of my peers and having my ears rubbed off in scrums. No selection by weight rather than age then. Irresponsible thugs with broken voices, cheesy breath and spotty faces enjoyed the temporary power that a few years' start gave them over their feebler, downy colleagues. Alas, I chose the more shameful path of anonymity, suppressing my outrage at a system of sanctioned bullying till more mature years. Cowardice and courage: how misleadingly those terms are used to undermine any shred of confidence a frail schoolchild can develop in an evil environment.

~

By the time my parents had removed me from this malignant influence and the men of the church who upheld it, I had acquired a very wary opinion of the establishment. I retain it yet.

It is possible to foster an entirely different attitude amongst schoolchildren. Emily and Morwenna both boarded. In an enlightened Dunedin school our children were accorded older girls as mentors to whom they could turn for help. A mentoring system employs psychology entirely diametric to the fagging of British public schools. Mentor or fag? There is simply no choice in a civilised society. A caring and kindly atmosphere is vastly more enriching for all concerned than the sanctioned, even encouraged, exploitation of the young and weak by the powerful. I am sure that the young ladies and men ensuing from such an enlightened system have greater self-assurance *and courage* than the twisted misfits that survived the great British public school boarding traditions.

It wasn't till much later that I read Thomas Hughes' nineteenth-century classic, *Tom Brown's Schooldays*. I was particularly interested in the preface of a later edition, where the author responds to the reception his work had received and, in particular, to the subject of bullying. A long letter he quotes from 'FD' eloquently sums up a problem that was to plague English public schools for another century.

I blame myself for not having earlier suggested whether you could not, in another edition of 'Tom Brown' or another story, denounce more decidedly the evils of bullying at schools...

A boy may have moral courage, and a fine organised brain and nervous system. Such a boy is calculated, if judiciously educated to be a great, wise and useful man; but he may not possess animal courage; *and one night's tossing, or bullying, may produce such*

an injury to his brain and nerves that his usefulness is spoiled for
life... A groom who tried to cure a shying horse by roughness and
violence would be discharged as a brute and a fool. A man who
would regulate his watch with a crowbar would be considered
an ass. But the person who thinks a child of delicate and nervous
organization can be made bold by bullying is no better.

He can be made bold by healthy exercise and games and sports;
but that is quite a different thing. And even these games and sports
should bear some proportions to his strength and capacities...

Why should the laws of civilization be suspended for schools?
Why should boys be left to herd together with no law but that of
force or cunning? What would become of society if it were consti-
tuted on the same principles? It would be plunged into anarchy
in a week.

What an insight, FD! In retrospect, I can now see how I was part
of those anarchistic tendencies.

I will not open the door for you because you wear a prefect's
tie. I will hear, but not heed, the message of those modulated tones
that you project over that massive lectern bible. I will not conform
to your expectations, and I will be subversive. Paradoxically, when
I leave here for the real world, I will not be inspired to join the
university demonstrations and follow the denim and kaftan-toting
leaders of my own generation against the conservatism of my elders.
I have glimpsed the worst excesses of my generation and I have little
faith that they can offer any improvement over the old guard.

I suspect that this is the insight that propels many ex-public
schoolboys. Those with the courage of their convictions will perhaps
tend to an Orwellian model of individual protest to engineer change
and rail against human injustice, rather than rally to the cries of
rent-a-mob. They will be suspicious of any form of authority, unless
it was thrust upon them at a tender age and gave them a lifelong
taste for its abuse.

~

Physical courage is present in some as of right, in some it is determined by a lack of imagination. For many it comes as a consequence
of character: mind over matter. The requirements are a supportive
and non-judgemental upbringing. He who is loved can love himself

and love others. From love comes confidence and from confidence, courage.

The ultimate use of courage is to secure justice… and to TB-test stags approaching the rut in marginal facilities.

This facetious interruption of childhood reveries raises a question seldom discussed by practising vets, or indeed farmers and others working with animals; it comes as second nature to them. We all have jobs to do around potentially dangerous animals. It is a matter of training and facilities that enable us to work with a minimum of danger. There is no room for heroics with a 600-kilo bull. It matters not whether you are a strapping 100-kilo prop forward or a fifty-kilo woman; brain, not brawn will be required. Odds of one-in-ten may be acceptable to a hero, but a vet has to be on the job every day. It has been said of another profession, 'There are old soldiers and there are bold soldiers, but there are no old, bold soldiers'.

Nevertheless, accidents do happen. I will never again TB-test stags in marginal facilities. They have very hard heads, even when the antlers have been removed. They push powerfully. When they start working their heads from side to side, you never know when they're going to stop. The owner, who told you how quiet they were, seems to have no idea what to do. Once cornered, twice shy. I just haven't got the guts to get back in the pen again. I know it's going to cost you more, and Daryl did some last month without any sedatives, but I'll just have to sedate them first, thank you very much.

CHAPTER THIRTY-FIVE

CHANGE, SUCCESS AND FAILURE

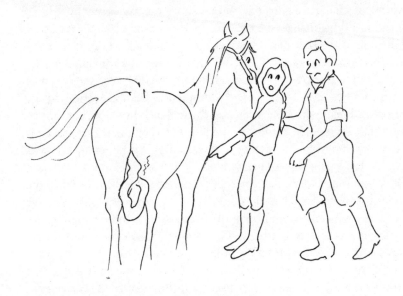

It has been remarked that in this modern world the average person should anticipate at least eight career changes through his working life. This magic number crops up in many unsubstantiated forms. London's inhabitants should know that when they drink from the tap, eight people will, on average, have preceded them in quaffing the recycled contents of the artesian wells of the Thames Basin. The average man or woman can anticipate the joys of eight sexual partners in a lifetime. Although I concede that this is a more variable figure, depending whether you defer towards the statistical analysis of *The Inquisitive Nerd* or *Cosmo-smut*, and that certain career choices would stretch the concept of 'the average' beyond meaning in this context.

The first person who drinks that glass of water from the Thames Water Supply Authority, is not materially different from the last.

If the first has superseded eight others, what of the eighth? Ah, statistics!

For some, a career change would be as memorable as my relationships example but, for the vast majority, change creeps up on them as insidiously, as innocuously as that recycled water. Career change doesn't necessarily leave us all at sixes and sevens.

From the day he or she qualifies, a veterinarian is on a constant spiral of change. There may be no more exams except for those seeking additional post-graduate qualifications, but the cycle of learning must continue. It is sobering to look back at our veterinary textbooks of the early 1970s. What was then encompassed in one handy volume now spills into several tomes. The seventies vet was at the end of an era where, with confidence, he could stride onto a farm and deal with whatever was thrown at him – dog, cat, horse, cow, sheep, pig. He could be relied upon to cope in these disparate areas of veterinary medicine with reasonable competence. It was a nice feeling. In ignorance is bliss. Thirty years later and even a small-animal expert may refer a skin or orthopaedic case on to the relevant specialist. That old school report lacked foresight. We have moved away from the polymath 'Renaissance man' model to an era where it now *is* a virtue to know more and more about less and less. For the animal-owning public the results may be better, but the costs are proportionately greater. In my opinion it is a major shame if a high-tech and expensive solution is offered for a patient without the low-tech alternative, which may be the only one that the owner can afford.

So I think back to the tips that as a youth I gleaned from the older practitioners who taught me. One of the commonest injuries to dogs, one that they share with footballers, is rupture of the cruciate ligament in the knee joint (or stifle as it is more accurately referred to in four-legged animals). The cruciate in fact comprises two ligaments in the centre of the stifle joint which permit the thigh bone (femur) to hinge on the shin bone (tibia), yet at the same time prevents the two bone ends from sliding on each other. Because the two ligaments cross over, the Latin term cruciate was applied by the early anatomists (Edinburgh graduates rejoice!). If one of the ligaments is torn, the joint becomes unstable, the dog cannot put weight on the leg and, if nothing is done, the unusual wear eventually damages the joint, setting up an irreversible arthritis.

It never pays to ignore the healing power of nature. Many injuries heal without intervention, perhaps not to perfection, but to an acceptable level. This is not generally the case with ruptured cruciates and many untreated dogs limping round the streets attest to this. They have three other legs, so generally they manage, but there is pain involved with arthritis and laissez faire can hardly be condoned.

For the vets of Miss Jericho's pre-war era a simple solution was to strap the stifle with a firm support of sticking plaster for a couple of weeks, perhaps injecting some of the dog's own blood into the joint. Thus immobilised, the damaged tissues could scar up and help support the joint, even if the ligaments themselves weren't repaired. This was better than doing nothing and in light dogs leading a fairly inactive life it is still a cheap and sometimes workable option.

But, as you may have guessed, there are at least eight ways of tackling a cruciate rupture. Since the last war surgical methods have been developed. Repairing the ligaments themselves is not an option for several reasons, but replacing them with fascia from surrounding tissues or even skin strips has become fairly standard. The stifle joint is opened and various tunnels drilled through the adjacent bones, depending on whose technique the surgeon prefers. The results are mostly favourable, even for active working dogs, perhaps partly due to the large amount of supporting scar tissue the body produces in response to the surgical insult. There is a simple elegance to such techniques, utilising existing tissues to create a structure that bio-mechanically simulates the damaged ligament.

Subsequently methods have evolved using synthetic implants, and even techniques requiring expensive equipment and specialist training. Great marketing, but certainly not practical for general purposes.

I have always derived satisfaction from treating injured dogs and the orthopaedic interventions required to restore them to health. Cats present less of a challenge, implicit in the maxim, 'as long as they're [that is, the two parts of the break] in the same room, the bone will knit'. Cats heal remarkably well, but not that well! For dogs and cats many bone fractures require stabilisation either externally, with casts or scaffolds, or internally, with pins, plates, wires or other devices. There are at least eight different ways to fix a fracture.

One day I was presented with Prince, a young black and white Border Collie who had fallen off a farm bike and fractured his femur close to his stifle joint. The x-rays showed the two broken ends of the bone over-riding each other. This was certainly something that required surgery but Prince's owner, Peter, was unwilling to spend the amount of money involved on a young and as yet unproven working dog. Prince was taken home and kept as quiet as it is possible to keep a six-month-old puppy.

A few weeks later he was walking around with a slight limp. Although plenty of three-legged dogs work sheep, I still envisaged that Prince's deformed leg was going to impede him, and I couldn't see him ever standing up to the rigours of working sheep without amputation. But Prince was a young dog and the fracture did heal. Quite often I saw him on the back of Peter's farm bike eager for work. Many years later I had the opportunity to take another x-ray of that old break. There was only a slightly abnormal curvature of the femur as a reminder of the fracture. Bone is not inert, as our familiarity with skeletal remains leads us to imagine. In the body it is a living tissue with the ability to remodel, and that is precisely what had happened. No surgery, no comfrey, no cider vinegar, no magnetic bandages, no colour therapy; though of course, if they had been used, success would have been attributed to them.

The boundaries are constantly explored and pushed with new knowledge and technology, but none would be possible without the healing power of nature and, given our belief in *our* interventions, often despite them or without them.

Why else do cats have *nine* lives?

~

A vet sees many strange and unusual events in the course of his career. The average punter with an interest in astronomy may have looked skywards on a clear night and seen a red dwarf. I confess that this is something of which I have only read. However, I have witnessed the castration of a Polish Dwarf in the bowels of the earth. Likewise a Flemish Giant. Before you are carried away by any Frankensteinian imagery I would have to confess that these are both breeds of rabbit, and I suppose that describing the cellar of the Victorian house where Craig had set up his surgery, in these terms, is a poetic exaggeration. Besides, castrating rabbits is scarcely thrilling fare. Once you have worked out a safe anaesthetic, the procedure can be completed in a calm and controlled fashion.

Castrating horses is another matter. The potential for drama is ever attendant, although modern anaesthetics have improved that aspect of the job. For much of my working life barbiturates injected into the jugular vein have been used successfully, but there is the drawback of a nasty local reaction to the drug should it be inadvertently injected into the tissues surrounding the vein, rather than the vein itself. If you are dealing with a frisky colt that is only partially broken-in, and you often are, the risks are obvious.

'Just hold still for a moment; you are going to feel a slight scratch', doesn't seem to work on horses. Humans can be conned into submitting themselves to all sorts of painful medical procedures. Not so your average horse. Pain infliction, or even the prospect of it, can invoke a violent response. Most horse vets have had a good kicking at some stage in their careers. For this reason a previous generation of horse vets had enviable roping skills and many had adopted the supreme technique of standing castration.

Approach your patient with a syringe loaded with local anaes-thetic. Inject it into the skin of the scrotum. Once you have placed that first vital bleb, it is possible to slowly work from the desensitised skin and infiltrate the whole area. The colt can be gelded while he indifferently chews on some nuts. The risks to the operator as that first bleb is placed are considerable. The firepower in those back legs is enormous. One false move may be your last. I have never worked in a practice where standing castrations were the norm, and so never felt pressured into using the technique. Throughout my life I have 'cheated' with barbiturates. The pressure did fall on a colleague who, newly graduated, went out with trepidation to his first standing castration. He had done the difficult bit and now approached the colt with scalpel in hand when it suddenly reared up. Inexperience took over and, in an attempt to evade the flailing hooves, he forgot about the scalpel poised in his hand. The horse landed on it, the sharp blade easily slicing right through the tensed abdominal muscles.

Anyone who has dealt with intestines will appreciate that they have a life of their own. The very peristaltic movements which drive food within them can impel them through the smallest hole.

Show them a gap and they will run for it. Gravity assists. Horrific war footage of soldiers clutching their escaping intestines is no exaggeration. A frightened horse has no incentive to do this and the end result of this sorry tale for my colleague was a scene of carnage. By the time the colt had trampled his intestines into the straw, the damage was irreversible and the poor animal was euthanased. I suspect that it was one very subdued vet who ventured out on his next foray to castrate a colt.

This tale of woe has always been at the back of my mind when I breeze up to another horse castration, but with barbiturates (or their modern equivalents), there is so much more control. It couldn't happen to me.

Every year Raewyn had a few colts for me to geld. It was a pleasant half-day outing. Her colts were well handled and she took no nonsense from them. This morning there were three to do. I had just finished the last one when the first was making its first staggering efforts to stand up. Raewyn was familiar with supervising recoveries from anaesthetics, ensuring that the worst effects of the drug had worn off before releasing the horses from their head collars and turning them loose to graze.

'John, I think there's something wrong.' There was a measure of anxiety underlying her usual calm competency. I glanced at colt number one. His intestines were sliding down his back leg. Very soon they would be in the dust. If ever I needed calm competency it was now.

'We're going to have to knock him out again,' I stated. Panicking is counter-productive and I have never felt that urge in such circumstances, but I did have a feeling of dread. The odds were stacked against a successful outcome. Raewyn was wonderful. She, too, would have had doubts, but she never let on.

Calmly she steadied the colt's head while I slipped in another dose of anaesthetic. Calmly she fetched a clean bucket and helped me to bathe the dust off the intestines and return them through the inguinal canal, the channel between the scrotum and abdominal cavity down which they had decided to eviscerate. This was not an easy procedure. The canal had to be enlarged, and yet it still required persistence and the dexterity of an octopus to finally overcome their obtuse writhing. It was with only partial relief that I put in the last sutures. Despite our care and attention to hygiene, horses are extremely prone to infections. There was still a grave risk of a fatal peritonitis, even with a heavy course of antibiotics. It would be several days before we knew his fate.

The colt recovered uneventfully. We had snatched victory from the bowels of defeat. Was this success or failure? Had I at the outset missed detecting a scrotal hernia, which would have alerted me to just this risk? In retrospect I felt not; I had had to enlarge the hole considerably merely to replace the intestines.

Such are the quandaries facing the veterinary clinician. Of all the thousands of successes, it is as much from the hundreds of mistakes and near misses that he learns. It is these that stick in his mind. We can only learn if we have a measure of self-doubt. Life never comprises endless chapters of glorious success.

CHAPTER THIRTY-SIX

LEAGUE OF NATIONS

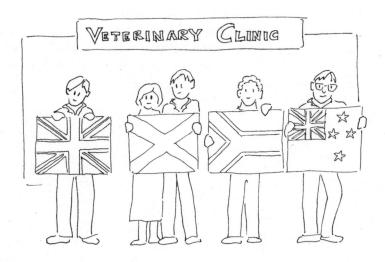

These days there is a shortage of New Zealand trained vets prepared to work in isolated rural communities. When Daryl and I sought to employ another vet the only suitable responses were from overseas applicants. Over the years we recruited a married couple, both Edinburgh graduates, and later a South African. Daryl, as the sole New Zealand vet, was starting to feel isolated. We are the products of universities from around the world and as a team we like to think that this gives us a collective strength, enabling us to tackle problems from our different perspectives. It also makes for interesting cultural observations.

From university days I have been aware of the unique cultural differences that mark us out. On my first day I had befriended a Welsh lad who most probably said something like, 'Hello, boyo, and where are you from?' Richard was raised in a Welsh-speaking family from South Wales. It was miraculous to hear him conversing rapidly over the phone with his family. Welsh was his first language, but that meant English was his second, and he good-naturedly fielded the teasing that was the inevitable consequence. A placid and sunny disposition frequently accompanies disarming gullibility, and Richard was no exception.

'Hey man, it says on the notice board that this meeting we're going to is at the Grosvenor Hotel, do we know how to get there?'

It reads innocuously, but Grosvenor is a word seldom encountered in the English language outside of its association with hotels. Few of us will ever encounter a grosvenor in full regalia during our dull little lives. There were obviously no Grosvenor hotels in Pontypridd, or Richard would not have pronounced it as Gros Veenor. It's not as though we would have pronounced Pontypridd correctly, but that is beside the point. He had said it to a group of like-minded friends and we instantly took up the challenge. We had him.

'Never mind, Richard,' said I, carefully borrowing his extreme rendition, 'We'll ask where the Gros Veenor is when we get into Chester.'

Somehow Richard ended up in the passenger seat on that journey, an ideal position from which to seek directions from some unsuspecting member of the public.

'Here's someone we can ask where the Grus Veeenor is,' said Tony eagerly. As we discussed the venue amongst ourselves the distortion had become monstrous. We pulled up beside an old man with a walking stick. Dutifully Richard wound down his window and politely made his request.

'Please can you tell us where the Grus Veeenor Hotel is?' The Welsh accent further elaborated the mutated name.

'I've lived here all my life and never heard of anything like that.'

Richard stuck to the task of diligently and insistently, attempting to prise the information from an increasingly puzzled old man. By this stage repressed giggles from the rest of the car's occupants were evolving into irrepressible snorts. Richard turned round from his difficult conversation in amazement. We were right opposite the Grosvenor Hotel.

'Look man, there! Across the road. The Grosvenor Hotel,' said

Tony, taking emphatic care to enunciate the vowels correctly and silence the central consonants.

Richard, as ever, was quick on the uptake. After apologising to the involuntary scapegoat he rounded on the rest of us in vulgar terms: 'You [adjective] bastards', was all he could say to general uproar, including his own.

~

The music of language is fascinating. A Welshman, if asked the difference between 'here's', 'ears' and 'years' will supposedly claim that there is none. Likewise for New Zealanders 'here' and 'hair', 'ear' and 'air', 'ferry' and 'fairy' are pairs of homonyms. E is invariably long, a long A an impossibility, and a short A is often rendered the same as a short E. It can cause problems, as this faithfully recorded conversation over a radio telephone will illustrate:

'John, can you go to Alley Beard at ---?'

'Was that Alley? I can't find an A Beard on the farm location map.'

'Alley's' initials, for which I was hunting, were in fact L E. 'Alley' was known by his second name, Elliott – Elly for short. Transposing A's and E's can be very confusing. We still had to solve the Beard/Baird part, but within half an hour I was on my way. It would have been churlish to have said, 'Oh, you mean Elliot Baird', but sometimes I am churlish, so that is precisely what I did say. Afterwards we had a good laugh about it and the ex-pats attempted to give Daryl and other members of the staff a decent mauling. The trouble is, they just aren't interested – a major cultural gulf. Kiwis couldn't give a stuff about mangling the language as long as they're winning the rugby. In that respect they're as bad as the Scots and Welsh. Since I am now a fully paid up member of the club, good manners behove me to desist from my Kiwi homonym phobia and so I wander around repeating to myself: 'sheared, shared; cheery, cherry; steer, stair; Elliot, Alliot; Beard, Baird.' My life would be easier if only I could cease spelling words in my head. 'Clarence, Clarance.'

Chris Clarence was one of our deer farming clients. As used to be usual in New Zealand – until the combination of thieves, cellphones and telephone directories put paid to the practice – his name was proudly displayed on his mail box at the entrance to the farm: C & T CLARENCE. I got to know Chris reasonably well after several seasons of develvetting and TB-testing his deer. He was pleasant company and a successful farmer. I had always been intrigued by the P CLARANCE mail box beside the driveway of the house across the road, directly opposite his, and commented about the coincidence.

'Oh, that's where my father lives,' he enlightened me.

'But Chris, why are the two names spelt differently then?' I asked, unaware that I was grossly transgressing the normal rules of grammar with my carelessly phrased question, until I wrote it down just now.

'They aren't, are they?'

Although I informed him that they were, the ENCE and ANCE mail boxes remained on the road for another five years, until the whole family moved to another district carrying their monuments to dyslexia with them.

Sheep farmers will tell you that there is more individual variation within breeds than between them. Working within a league of nations, as our vets have been described, I cannot but fail to agree. There are national characteristics, but the same virtues and vices are present in us all. However, tea room conversations would be less interesting were we to accede to this homily.

~

'Darling, do you think it's safe to air your prejudices like this? You could offend a lot of people.'

'No, it isn't safe and I realise that it reflects sadly on me. I should be linguistically liberal and accept that our language is a living thing, constantly evolving. What I can't understand is why we need to alter pronunciations and word meanings and spellings for the sake of effect or novelty and cause confusion where there needn't be. Least of all I cannot abide changes supposedly implemented for reasons of logic.'

'Alright, alright. I know where you're heading now.'

'Yes, our New World cousins. At least the colonials haven't ridden roughshod over the language and changed all the spellings.'

'But they retained some of the old spellings and it was the English who altered them subsequently.'

'Yes, I can't argue with that. But let me have one last rant. Folks out there should realise what has been happening to their language on the frontiers of science. We used to have wonderful words with classical derivations. I know I was no Latin scholar, but I do think the language should retain echoes of our linguistic history. Changing the spelling of oestrus to estrus, foetus to fetus, dropping the "a" from haemoglobin to become hemoglobin: it all seems neat and tidy until the next generation comes along and starts mispronouncing these words based upon the new spellings.'

'It's your age dear.'

It is not possible to win every argument, but honour dictates that we stand up for what we feel is right. With some issues feelings countermand logic. Language is one of them, but heaven forbid I be categorised as a fuddy-duddy for my beliefs.

CHAPTER THIRTY-SEVEN

DISMANTLING THE BARRIERS OF DISTASTE

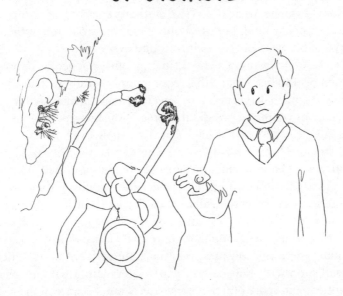

'Go on, John, have a listen to this dog's chest.' Mr Betts was encouraging me to broaden my veterinary education. He took the stethoscope out of his hairy ears. Was I expected to insert the globby, off-white, plastic ear pieces with their streaks of wax directly into my own ears? The answer was yes. My veterinary education had taken a new twist and, from being a naturally fastidious person who disdained sharing a cup with even my own family members, I was now to embark on a process of desensitisation. True, Miss Jericho had pushed the boundaries too far, but in time the mind can be conditioned to over-ride feelings of revulsion, and looking back it seems that a large part of a vet's training involves dismantling these natural barriers of distaste.

There is a peril in this. The instincts to avoid sharing body fluids, and be squeamish about torn flesh and blood, body wastes and stinking corpses are an evolutionary protection mechanism. They minimise our exposure to noxious organisms. For vets the hazards from disease are greater than the risks of physical injury.

Diseases communicable from animals to man are designated zoonoses. *Brucella abortus*, the bacterium that claimed the life of Mike, and many other vets of his era, is a classic example; but vets are regularly exposed to a cocktail of potentially dangerous and even life-threatening micro-organisms. We can pay attention to personal hygiene, wear protective clothing, splash the appropriate disinfectants around, but inevitably situations arise where there is unavoidable risk. Zoonoses lurk round every corner.

Picture in your mind a cow urinating onto a concrete slab with the sun behind her. I make this request not for aesthetic reasons. In this light golden droplets can be seen to sparkle as they arch up and out, encompassing a considerable area. Now imagine that you are truncated to chest height and placed a couple of feet from where that stream of urine hits the slab. This is precisely the position of a dairy worker in a modern herringbone milking shed. His face is regularly exposed to urine droplets and vapour. If the cow is a Leptospirosis carrier, she will be shedding lethal little leptospires in her urine capable of being absorbed through mucous membranes such as lips and eyes. Should he contract the disease he will develop flu-like symptoms and progress to a state where if he isn't dead, he will soon wish that he was. Early intervention with antibiotic treatment will spare him the worst effects but, because of the vague early symptoms, the connection may not be made. A disease that can be relatively innocuous in one species can be devastating in another.

In the late 1990s a tourist to New Zealand harboured a previously unrecorded bacterium in his or her intestines. From the sewage ponds of Christchurch it is speculated that seagulls strewed the infection across the immaculate pastures of Canterbury and launched a new disease on the livestock industry. *Salmonella Brandenburg* is an interesting variant of the usual strains of salmonellae that we encounter in New Zealand in that it is predisposed to seek out the pregnant uterus and cause abortion. Sheep are at greatest risk, and when the first wave of infection reached Southland our clinic was deluged with aborted lamb foetuses brought in to us by local farmers anxious to identify the reason for their losses.

Dabbling in the cold, smelly and slimy little carcases to retrieve samples of stomach contents, heart blood, brain and placenta is one of the most disgusting jobs imaginable. Even so it is possible to suppress the distaste in the interests of science. On the shiny stainless steel table of our post-mortem room, wearing double gloves, gumboots, waterproof overalls and with plenty of water and disinfectant, we felt in control. The risk of infection, although those carcases were hooching with pathogenic organisms, was relatively slight.

It was a different matter when, the following season, *Salmonella Brandenburg* started showing up in cattle. When a full-term calf dies inside a cow it may not be expelled immediately. Natural lubricating fluids that ease the passage of the calf dry up. The cow herself starts to sicken and weaken, and the calf rots and expands with gas. The poor unsuspecting vet is on his way again.

As I have described before, rotten calvings are not unusual for vets. One rotten calving is much like another. At midnight by torchlight, how are we to know that we are witnessing the manifestations of a hitherto unrecorded disease? Calving that cow as she squats down, straining an aerosol broth of salmonellae into your grimacing face, merely inches away, is virtually guaranteed to overwhelm the strongest immune system and give licence to those bacteria to colonise your body.

That year three of our staff went down with severe dysenteric symptoms confirmed as *Salmonella Brandenburg*. Recovery to full health can take months.

Fortunately the faeces of healthy ruminants are largely recycled grass containing a large proportion of chlorophyll, a natural deodorising chemical. The large-animal vet's task is not as unpleasant as some may imagine. On a cold winter's day there is no quicker way to warm the hands then to indulge in a spot of pregnancy testing. The use of scanning machines has obviated this advantage, but there are compensations.

For a phenomenal capital outlay we obtained an ultrasonic scanning device that could be of use in many species. As a rectal probe, using heaps of lubricant, we can ascertain pregnancy in cows, sheep, deer and horses. For dogs and cats it can be placed on the belly for the same purpose – rather as an ultrasound scan for human pregnancy.

One of our vets had been out all day scanning hinds. The scanner's probe, basically a modified human machine, had been well protected with black silage tape. I retrieved it from its shelf by the back door and hurriedly wiped it clean. I needed it to scan Mrs Dickens' immaculate white Maltese Terrier. Was she pregnant? She sat, a picture of groomed perfection, on the consulting room table. Mrs Dickens, as elegant and well-groomed as her charge, chatted as I applied the lubricant to that precious tummy. It took some time, as is the case when there is nothing to find. I angled the probe in different directions.

'I'm sorry, Susan, but I can't make her pregnant. Oops, it looks as if we have another problem here.'

I was looking at a large dark pool of faecal matter spreading over the table and already tinting those lustrous locks. It was also on my hand and the sleeve of my coat.

'That's strange,' observed Mrs Dickens, 'she has been the picture of health recently. Perhaps she's nervous.' She glared peevishly at the innocent-looking dog.

After careful examination, I had drawn a blank.

'Perhaps you're right. Look, her temperature's OK and I can't find anything else wrong. I doubt that there is a problem. It hasn't even got an offensive smell to it. Let me know if you do have any concerns.' And then the truth dawned.

Surreptitiously I set the probe aside and guided her to the door. When I returned an even bigger pool had run out of the tape protecting the head of the probe. A pool comprising three parts lubricant and one part deer faeces makes a horrible mess.

Words were said about cleaning up equipment after you have used it. Sometimes jokes about leaving you in the proverbial aren't appreciated and the hoary old one as to whether I was sure it was a Maltese and not a Shih Tzu (say it quickly) was trotted out, but eventually I saw the funny side. There had been worse messes to clean up.

CHAPTER THIRTY-EIGHT

SOUTHLAND'S SECRETS

The hours when the mind is absorbed by beauty are the only hours when we really live, so that the longer we can stay among these things so much the more is snatched from inevitable Time.

Richard Jefferies

Fly west to the mountain fastness of Fiordland; north, up the mighty folds of the Southern Alps; glide east from there over the arid plateaux of Otago; east again where the cool, damp forests of the Catlins enfold a mysterious coast; to the south the bulk of Stewart Island, unspoilt nature within its sparkling shores. Large lakes wash the feet of rugged mountains. Te Anau, a veritable inland sea, its three western arms twining under remote peaks; glittering Manapouri with its scatter of islands, tentacles probing a jagged wilderness; narrow and moody Hauroko, deepest of them all, claiming a Maori princess in a secret island cave. This is the unparalleled heritage to which Southlanders enthusiastically lay claim. Here they can hunt, tramp, fish, ski and wonder as they inhale the cool freshness of primordial forests. Here was our new playground.

Was it the pure air, healthy lifestyle and good food of Southland that had gifted Viv and me our two fine daughters? No matter, after years of indignities and hospital tests we had been blessed within a few months of our arrival.

Before we were long in Southland we had completed some of the great walks, tramped before the rock ramparts of the Darren Mountains, looked down on the crevasses and moraines of the Dart Glacier, and seen the secretive rock wrens amongst their home in the boulder fields of the Rees. Once again we were amazed by the sheer botanical diversity of New Zealand's largely endemic flora: from forest floors carpeted with ferns, mosses and lichens to vegetable sheep, sentries on the high screes. Once more we were 'hutting' in places of wild isolation.

And so we have come to another spiritual home, far removed from the soft greens of the Anglo-Saxon dream-world where I commenced my journey. Here among the sombre mountain beech forests a harsh realm of delicate beauty unfolds. A sea of tussock grass extends between scattered islands of ancient trees, and gives way to the alpine herb fields we will soon ascend. But let us linger awhile and look up to the snow and rock above. The red-gold of the morning sun already catches the topmost peaks. A day of promise is unfolding, but here is still a half-world of roiling mists. Where the trees enclose the damper air above a rushing stream, the gnarled branches of the ancient ones are draped in hanging lichens: *goblin forest*. The poverty of the thin and sour soils, the drenching rains and heavy snows demand they strive for a hundred years or more to attain even the modest height of a man. Their struggle confers character and nobility, as it does to all those who emerge dignified, if battle-scarred, from great hardships.

The air is washed in this damp climate to coolest purity. Far to the west the ridges rake into a wild and lonely part of the Tasman Sea...

Perhaps we shall hear the wild and joyous cry of the kea bent on another day of mischievous playfulness, perhaps merely the gentle soughing of a damp wind but, as yet, there is a blanket of expectant silence.

The clank of a billy reminds us of that first luxurious draught of hot tea, and recalls our party to a companionable breakfast in the smoky hut. Hunched over a rude wooden table, knobbly with candle wax, our murmured conversations vaporise in the cool air.

We are on the Dusky Track, a testing route through the heart of Fiordland. It twists over the Main Divide from the head of Lake Hauroko to Dusky Sound, first place of landfall for Captain Cook on his visit of 1773; still pristine and remote. Then it doubles back over another high pass to the West Arm of Lake Manapouri, a trip of seven or eight days. Away to the east and over the ranges, where the bush wilderness is tamed to farmland, Cedric, a successor to Boris, romps in a rough bush paddock on Jean Sinclair's farm.

The track, such as it is, meanders round and through swamps, over fallen trees, and up and down vertiginous glaciated valley sides. The climate is bleak and predominantly wet. Tramping it involves considerable physical effort, but the rewards are immense.

At the end of the second day our party of four, warmly ensconced in our sleeping bags, were enjoying the cosy satisfaction of full stomachs and safe shelter. We relaxed in the gathering gloom and, by ten o'clock or so, we were all fast asleep. And then, somehow, by a mechanism it would be hard to define, we were aware of a *presence*. A sly, secretive presence. It could have been a rat, but the rustles and clanks became gradually more insistent. Our curiosity was aroused most of all by a faint, rhythmic, brushing sound.

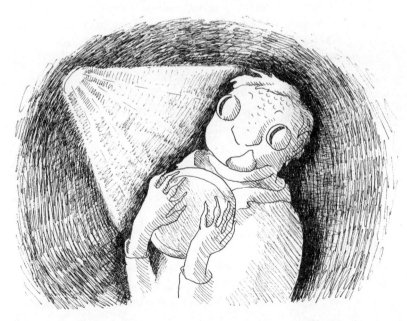

I flashed on my torch and there, frozen in the beam, was a wild-looking individual. His plate was next to his face, his tongue which had been employed licking out its contents, now slowly traversed his upper lip. This nocturnal image of reptilian furtiveness was to lodge in our minds. Henceforth he was the Gecko.

To my offered apology and greeting he responded not one word.

How could he have found the hut in the dark? It was a moonlit night, but he appeared to have no torch. This was country where it was easy to put a foot wrong and get lost, even in broad daylight. It was no isolated event; the same pattern was repeated at subsequent huts. The mysterious Gecko was imbued with almost supernatural qualities, at least in my mind. My companions were also intrigued. And still he never spoke a word, even when spoken to directly.

At last we saw him writing in the hut book, and seized an opportune moment to learn more of this strange apparition. Ah! He was German. That would explain the lack of communication. As luck would have it, at the next hut there were some other Germans. We were relived to see that he did possess a functioning larynx, for he spoke with them, albeit briefly. They, too, seemed fazed by the eccentricity of the Gecko. Later they told us that this was no ordinary German, in fact they were keen to point out that he spoke Swiss-German with an English accent, and that he was, in fact, English.

Over the days, we slowly gained his confidence and had limited conversations with him. I found out that he was an engineer who had spent many years working in Switzerland. His home town was Liverpool. In my mind he was immediately and inevitably linked to the newspaper familiar to all Liverpudlians. Here before me was the Liverpool Gecko!

It is at times like these, in the remotest parts of the world, that you realise what a small place it can be. The Liverpool Gecko, as it turned out, was a product of my old school. The English public school system had struck again.

Regrettably, we found it impossible to converse effectively with our reptilian associate. He was a true eccentric. But wild individual-ists are not the norm in these isolated huts and, usually, the people who tramp the back-blocks are sociable and communicative. They share a love of their surroundings and that cheerful spirit required to overcome adversity.

The tribulations of the day are leavened by conversing with such company, and by perusal of the hut books. There, amid the coffee stains and squashed sandflies, the weary traveller will encounter much dross, but occasional pearls from others who have shared the same travails: mud, snow, rain, floods and sandflies. Who could resist this gem, gleaned from the book at the Kintail hut?

The Dusky Simulator
Try the Dusky Track at home without an expensive aeroplane ride! Here's all you have to do...

Dig a large hole (over your head) in your back lawn. Fill the bottom of the hole with quicksand and then top up with water – just enough to make it level with the lawn so it looks like a shallow hole.

Tip in a bucket of eels, five buckets of ice cubes and set the garden sprinkler going at one end.

Now forget you've dug the hole and come home later that night with no flashlight and maintaining good speed walk straight into the hole. Remember to flail your arms about uselessly as you fall in. Get out under the sprinkler and repeat a hundred times.

Score a point for every time you don't swear.

Well done! You've just done a day on the Dusky Trail – go inside and try to light some soggy firewood with some wet matches and make a well-deserved cup of tea!

Such anonymous self-deprecating humour encapsulates much of what is best about the human spirit. This extract was owed more than an ephemeral life, I thought, as I copied it into my diary: a wider readership than the few hardy souls who would be lucky enough to time their tramp during the few brief months of its display.

~

Today, as I look to the west I can see the mountains of Fiordland and I am comforted to know of the glorious wilderness that lies beyond. Some untrammelled corners of our crowded planet, untouched by the clumsy developments of man, are essential for our collective sanity. Even when I am too old or frail to seek their sanctuary, my spirit will seek their solace.

As I muse, I cannot suppress a vision from my childhood.

A bright night of full moon. A night of fresh clarity after rain. A cool breeze tears apart the ragged clouds, revealing a scene of unearthly beauty. Below us lie the ancient oak woods, the very ones that clutch that cow-wheat in their mystic depths. But here the silver light bathes the slate roof of the stone farmhouse. My parents, my brother and I stand transfixed, in awe of this rare moment of sublimity. Through the racing gaps of light and shadow, across the Conway valley, the peaks of Snowdonia parade across the western sky: the Glyders, Tryfan, the notch of the Nant Ffrancon and, directly opposite, the dark bulk of the Carnedds. These are places we had enjoyed together, had come to know and love. But for my father this would have been a moment of added poignancy; invoked by Tryfan's rocky summit. On those steep crags he had rock-climbed with his elder brother on their last shared leave. Precious time together: release from the horrors of war.

As my vision is replayed, divine music, owing nothing to any man-created god, ebbs and eddies, washes and flows, salving my mind. This is music that I have shared with those I love, perhaps the adagio from Mendelssohn's atmospheric 'Scottish': music to transform the spirit, music to balm the soul. And again, another visit to this Celtic dreamscape, plunged in moonlight, may suit less structured perfection: more passionate intensity. Music that strives hauntingly and, for brief, searing moments, captures the essence of wild ecstasy. For this *I* would choose the slow, glittering silver of a Bax symphony, the moment where the dissonant horns reach for the impossible. Music conveys rapture where words fail. It is but one of many joys in this world.

~

Being a vet and having such an interesting career has been immensely satisfying and challenging. However, a career is but a part of life, part of one section of the journey. I confess to a troubled respect for those individuals motivated entirely by their profession. There has to be a balance. Becoming a vet is no passport to happiness.

If I could impart any wisdom it would be that it is essential to develop other passions. Furnish your mind; there can be little joy in an empty room. Love; enjoy your family and, for your children, sow the seed; appreciation comes from within. Nurture those spiritual homes. If such is your inspiration, go to the hills from whence cometh your help (an ancient wisdom). Treasure unspoilt environments. Tune in to the beauty and emotion of great music; search for that which speaks to your soul. Immerse yourself in the inventiveness of inspired prose. Travel and learn from other cultures. Delve into history, and understand the guiding principles of civilisation, its very future depends on a motivated and informed populace.

There are more important things in life than Fru-Fru, even if our love for her enshrines an important aspect of our humanity.